DISEASES OF THE RESPIRATORY
and
DIGESTIVE SYSTEM OF CHILDREN

by

Dr. L. Rousseau
Dr. Fortier-Bernoville

TRANSLATED FROM THE ORIGINAL FRENCH BY

Dr. Rajkumar Mukerji
M.A., L.H.M.S.

B. JAIN
Publishers (Pvt.) Ltd.

Price: Rs. 35.00

Published by

KULDEEP JAIN

for

B. Jain Publishers (P) Ltd.

1921, Chuna Mandi, St. 10th Paharganj,
New Delhi-110 055

Phones: 91-011-2358 0800, 2358 1100, 2358 1300
Fax: 91-011-2358 0471; Email: bjain@vsnl.com
Website: www.bjainbooks.com

Printed in India by
J. J. Offset Printers

ISBN : 81-7021-389-4
BOOK CODE : 2053

―――

This Translation is

DEDICATED

to

"Kuntala"

―――

CONTENTS

PREFACE

"Disease of the Digestive system of Children" is a translation of the article "Treatment Homoeopathique des troubles de 1' Apparel digestive et de la nutrition dans la premiere enhance" by Dr. Fortier – Bernoville, which was published in the journal **1' Homoeopathic Modern No.** 12, 15th June, 1934, and the second article "Diseases of the Respiratory system of children" is a translation of the article "1" Homoeopathic infantile dans less affection aigkues des voices respiratories" by A. L. Rousseau published in the same issue of the same journal. The third article is a summary of a lecture delivered by Dr. Fortier-Bernoville in the 1'Ecole francaise d'Homoeopathie on the 4th May, 1937. This translation was first published in the journal Hahnemannian Gleanings for its topographical interest, No. 12, December, 1972.

In these articles the readers will often meet with the words "Constitution & Temperament" and the word "Drainage", The words Constitution and Temperament as understood by the French homoeopaths are somewhat different to what we understand by them. Drainage is a word foreign to us. For the proper understanding of these terms I would ask my readers to go through my two books "Constitution and Temperament" and "What we must not do in Homoeopathy", published by Jain Publishers.

Chandarnagor
June, 1976   Rajkumar Mukerji

INTRODUCTION

This books needs an introduction because of the words like "Drainage", "Drainer", Tuberculinics", "Tubercular conditions" etc. which are new to the Homoeopaths of India. The drainage is one of the most important system of Homoeopathic treatment among the French homoeopaths. In short, drainage is nothing but the use of remedies having ephemeral action in order to help in the eliminatory functions of the antipsoric remedies. The helping remedies are generally the complementaries and antidotes of the principal basic remedy. The antidotes are used as an umbrella working as a check, in the too dangerous eliminatory functions of the basic drug, which may cause aggravation of the disease.

The word "tuberculinic" "tubercular conditions" have been introduced into homoeopathy by Dr. A. Nebel of Lausanne who made serious investigations on tuberculines. It is Dr. Nebel who says that "If the word Psora does not merit to be maintained only to honour the memory of Hahnemann, we may replace it with Tuberculinism".

Some explanations are required about the above two facts in order that the principle of drainage and canalisation and identity of tubercular condition with Psoric miasm may not be misunderstood by the readers of this little book. I have, therefore, given in the introduction the summary of two lectures of Dr. Fortier-Bernoville, one on "Identity of

Psora and tuberculinism" delivered in Glasgow (1936) and the other on principles of Drainage and Canalisation.

Identity of Psora with Tuberculinism

"If the name Psora does not merit to be maintained in order to honour the memory of Hahnemann, we replace it by the word tuberculinism". It is thus Dr. A, Nebel expressed himself in 1934. This opinion has become very much current among the French homoeopaths. It should be supported by 1. Clinic, 2. Laboratory works and 3. Homoeopathic therapeutics.

Let us see first of all what Psora of Hahnemann is?

It is according to the Master the most common, the most contagious and the most stubborn miasm. He called "itch" not only to lesions caused by Sarcopotes but also to all chronic, polymorphous eruptions which have the principal characteristic, when suppressed, of causing numerous and varied metastasis. He shows by the help of numerous documentaries that the Psora may be succeeded by "Suffocating catarrh, hydropsy, pleuresy, all sorts of cough and hemoptysis, meningitis, ascites, hydrocele, jaundice, deafness, diabetes, haemorrhoids etc." The genius of Hahnemann has been singularly illuminated by the researches of Richet, Vidal and A. Lumiere.

What do we mean by tuberculous virus according to the works of modern biologists?

After the discovery by Koch the bacilli of Tuberculosis which Villemin foresaw, numerous kinds of alcohol or acid resistants have been discovered. At that time, one did not admit the existence of tuberculosis until and unless, Koch's bacilli were detected by the microscope in the sputum. At present, the discovery of tubercular ultra-viruses, which are capable to cross through the placenta (Hauduroy, Arloing, Dufour) and cause contagion *in utero* (Calmette, Valtis, Negre, Boquet) has completely exploded the theory of Koch's bacilli. The importance of cuti-reactions which were then completely unknown has now become very important. Thus heredo-tuberculosis has become a reality like that of heredo-syphilis, which proves the theory of Psora.

We have then two theories: That of Psora and that of Tuberculinism. Now we will show their identity:

1. Clinical proofs.

The works of Bezacon and Jacquelin (Congress on Asthma, 1933), show the close relation of Asthma with tuberculosis. The children of asthmatics very often become tubercular or inversely. It is also seen that asthma develops in chronic tubercular patients cured or in persons having calcified cavities.

Poncet has long ago described a form of Rheumatoid arthritis of tubercular origin. Numerous forms of arthritis are now attributed to the tubercular viruses. It is this conception which has led to the use of Gold in cases of rheumatoid arthritis, with frequent success. Let us note that the reaction of Vernes-resorcine is very often positive in these affections.

The tubercular form of salpingitis has a tendency of becoming more important. Pure of gonorrheal forms are associated. Same thing is considered in appendicitis (Cancal tuberculosis).

Some good results are obtained by anti-tubercular treatment in several other diseases. Asthma with *Tuberculines* (Jacqueline), treatment of rheumatism by chrysotherapy, methilic antigene or allergine.

Kent has shown alternate states of dementia and tuberculosis. Some anxiety neurosis are also attributed to tuberculosis.

In endocrinal troubles, tuberculosis is of great importance with syphilis (Addison's disease, diabetes, Basedow's disease etc.)

Systematic study of personal hereditary antecedents in psoric patients proves, alternance of diseases, which shows that there is predisposition to tuberculosis.

2. Laboratory results

The cuti-reactions to *Tuberculines* are positive in 97% of cases in adults. Their intensity varies following anti-tubercular treatment by the application of diluted *Tuberculines*.

Vernes-resorcin reactions which are positive in tuberculosis in evolution, is positive in rheumatisms, which leads one to think that it is related to tuberculous infections.

Pulmonary radiography shows in almost all individuals more or less discrete and sclerosed lesions of chronic tuberculosis.

This last information is confirmed by the autopsies in course of which the extreme frequency of calcified tubercles are discovered.

3. Arguments from Homoeopathic therapeutics

It is first of all necessary to take some cases which will show us in our psoric patients, the foliation with tuberculosis. In such cases, the addition of a diluted *Tuberculine* to the treatment is indicated. We know, on the other hand, that in the majority of chronic assess, it is only after the use of a *Tuberculine* that we get final cure. The aggravation, almost constant in patients who are give *Tuberculine* at the beginning of the Treatment, had led Dr. Nobel to think that Psora was identical to tuberculinism. It is in order to avoid the aggravations, he found out his method of drainage. These aggravations, are seen in hypertensive, arteriosclerotic, arthritic, venous, uremic patients and in some patients having stones, eczema, urticaria. Thus the arthritic diathesis which seems to be on the antipodes of tuberculosis is on the contrary attenuated tuberculinic. These patients have hypercholesterinemia which is nothing but an exaggeration of the defense against the tuberculous virus. Instead of caseifying, the cause sclerosis. The parasitosis are also under the dependence of tuberculinic (intestinal worms, colibacillosis).

Finally if the Hahnemannian description of psora is compared with the pathogenesis of *Tuberculimum* one will be astonished to see the analogy of the important symptoms. Dr. Renard has besides shown that *Psorinum* and *Tuberculimum* are interchangeable.

Therefore Psora seems to us clearly the ensemble of hereditary tubercular manifestations.

How can we explain the identification of psora with tuberculinism?

J. Sedillot has explained the role of hepatic insufficiency causing different manifestations, which are apparently different and autonomous. He explains how the residues (nitrogenated) incompletely transformed by the weak liver are over-saturated in the blood serum where it flocculates either during a momentary overcharge of the liver (faulty diet), or during an anaphylactising cause (pollen, emotion etc). These flocculates are phagocytosed by the monocytes, which, not being able to divest themselves of their renal epithelial burden, are eliminated through points where congestion of blood favours the exudation. In babies it is the skin, the fragile barrier. It is very often irritated specially that of the orifices, causing oozing lesions which become secondarily infected and gives birth to oozing eczema. When later on the skin will become hard. we will find furuncles and urticarieas; then come different tropism's: asthma during the first bronchitis. Later on the favourite points of elimination will change and tropism's will be modified.

This hepatic deficiency, which remained undetermined to Sedill ot, seems to us to be the fact that foetus is contaminated by the tuberculous virus (Bernard). Because of the constant arrival during long months, of ultravirus into the liver through umbilical cord and vitelliness, and abnormal proliferation of the conjunctive tissues of that organ is caused, because it is the tissue (reticulo-endothelial) which is precisely meant to produce the monocytes which will phagocyte are the flocculates.

Thus we understand: 1. The identification of psora and tuberculinism. 2. Multiple psoric manifestations and their polymorphism.

In Summary

Psora is therefore the direct consequence of tubercular affection, very often hereditary, sometimes acquired in lower age.

Its characteristics are: 1. Alternance, 2. Endocrinal troubles, 3. Vago-sympathetic disturbances, 4. Troubles of tissue tonus, 5. Cutaneous tropism, 6. Parasitical tendency, 7. Predisposition to contagious diseases, 8. Suppurative tendency, 9. Troubles of mineralisation.

Tuberculinism seems therefore the primordial and primary cause of majority of chronic diseases. It is like a background canvas on which are projected the other secondary manifestations: trauma, shocks, emotional shocks, anaphylactic phenomena etc.

Finally I must add that Kent has called psora "Urschadiguna" i.e. the original sin of human being. As such we may describe and understand psora in a different manner. We call psora as the scourge of human civilization which is making man prone to all sorts of diseases. If the reader feels himself interested in my exposition of psora as the scourge of civilization, he may refer to my article "Homoeopathy in search of the total man" published in the Hahnemannian Gleanings, January, No. 1, 1970.

Now let me speak something about the Drainage and Canalisation as Dr. Fortier-Bernoville understands it.

Drainage and Canalisation in Homoeopathic therapeutics

It is to Dr. A. Nebel we owe the idea of Drainage and its corollary Canalisation, one of the most important principles of Homoeopathic therapeutics. Drainage was practiced since Hippocrates up to our time by Rademacher, by Hahnemann himself and finally by Burnett.

Definition

When we speak of drainage, we should distinguish well the

theory from the practice. In order not to run the risk of being reproached as builders of purely theoretical systems, we will speak here only of the results obtained from the practice of drainage and canalisation, the theory having, in our opinion, only explanatory value, of simple orientation.

However, we should give a theoretical definition of drainage before speaking about its practical application.

The theory of drainage is intimately bound with the idea of making the organism free from morbid energies. If we understand an organism as composed of many spheres, we will see that it is necessary to give one or more medicines acting simultaneously on the successive organic spheres.

But a single remedy, even highly diluted cannot always act in a sure and complete manner on all the spheres and generally the high dilutions help to obtain a superior action on the most subtle and higher planes, particularly on the sphere of sympatbetic system.

It is therefore necessary to help the *Similimum* by a judiciously selected remedy which is *Simile*.

It is said that in each pathological case there exists in Homoeopathy, a single *Similimum* and *Simile* and the first idea that comes to mind is to apply uniquely the *Similimum* with the exception of *Simile* remedies that seem to be palliatives.

In reality, very soon one understands that the rigorous

application of the *Similimum* remedy is not always followed and is not necessarily followed by an amelioration. If we can prepare the organism by the application of a remedy called satellite, or the remedy, which by analogy, has the symptoms culled from the patient, it happens very often that the *Similimum* may be applied afterwards WITHOUT AGGRA-VATION and it seems to act even more rapidly and more deeply.

THE THEORY OF DRAINAGE IS, THEREFORE, BEFORE ALL, A THEORY OF PURIFICATION OF THE INTOXICATED ORGANISM THAT SHOWS SYMPTOMS WHICH MAY BE CLASSIFIED ACCORDING TO THE SUCCESSIVE SPHERES OF THE ORGANISM AND THE DISAPPEARANCE OF THESE SYMPTOMS CANNOT BE CAUSED IN A COMPLETE AND RAPID MANNER BUT BY THE APPLICATION GENERALLY OF MANY REMEDIES SIMULTATNEOUSLY OR SUCCESSIVELY.

The theory of drainage is, therefore, a theory of purification. Besides, the term Drainage, so often used in surgery, is understood better when one is only on the material plane. There is no doubt that when there is a suppuration in the organism, it is necessary to eliminate the formed pus, except in some cases where it is possible to obtain a complete resorption.

It is therefore, necessary to purify the organism of the patient by eliminating the toxin. It is necessary to drain.

But drainage considered from the point of view of

practice is much more important than from the point of view of theory. THE DRAINAGE IS BEFORE ALL A PRACTICE JUSTIFIED BY RESULTS. The theory of drainage like all theories is seducing but it is rather easy. We need not find out up to what point it may be true according as one represents it in such and such a manner, but it is necessary before all to insist on the fact that it is fecund and that this fecundity is the only justification that we require. THE PRACTICE OF DRAINAGE CONSISTS IN FOLLOWING OR IN PRECEDING THE PRINCIPAL INDICATED REMEDY BY THE APPLICATION OF ONE OR MORE SATELLITE REMEDIES WITH THE AIM OF FACILITATING THE TOXIC ELIMINATION IN A GIVEN MORBID STATE, TO CHECK MEDICINAL AGGRAVATION AND TO OBTAIN MORE RAPID AND SURE RESULTS.

Experience shows that the systematic and rational application of antidotes and complementaries of Hahnemann, side by side with the principal remedy forms the real key to the practice of drainage. It is thus that Dr. Nebel has shown to us by attractive examples the value of drainage. He has, for example shown to us that before *Calcarea carbonica* is applied to a patient who has its symptoms, one may obtain good results, and can check all aggravations in tubercular patients, by giving at first *Pulsatilla* which is a real drainer of *Calcarea carbonica*.

In other cases where there is an acute and temporary febrile condition *Belladonna* may be a satellite of *Calcarea carbonica* and which is necessarily indicated before the ground remedy. Sometimes the satellite may be *Dulcamara* or *Chamomilla*.

Let us now speak of *Canalisation*.

We should also understand Canalisation from the theoretical and practical point of view.

From the theoretical point of view THE PRINCIPLE OF CANALISATION RESTS ON THE IDEA OF THE LOCAL ELECTIVE ACTION OF MOST OF THE REMEDIES USED IN HOMOEOPATHY.

It appears then that the principle of Canalisation is a corollary of the principle of Drainage. To canalise means to DIRECT THE ACTION OF REMEDY IN SPACE AND AS WELL AS IN TIME. Canalisation consists in the real study of the physiopathologic action of remedies.

To canalise is to direct the effects of a medicinal substance and to orient its action. When we speak of the local elective action of a remedy, it is necessary to speak precisely here, that most of the remedies may have, from spatial point of view, some elective actions, either on the tissues, on the organs, or on the topographic region oriented along the nervous system or very often according to a metameric segmentation. There exists, therefore, three kinds of local elective actions which rule canalisation. In practice, to give a satellite which will have for aim to canalise and orient the effects of principal remedy; that action becomes naturally in part a real check. When we give to a patient a dose of the high dilution of *Sulphur* according to the symptoms (while the patient has also the tendency to suppuration), we may do good to the general condition, but at the same time we may have some dangerous local effects, by increasing the tendency to suppuration. If on the contrary, we know how to canalise the too centrifugal, violent and general action of *Sulphur,* on such and such parts of the organism, we will surely obtain good action of this remedy. *Nux vomica* for small intestines, *Aloe* for the rectum etc. In this case we may say that these different remedies are the Canaliser of *Sulphur,* because they canalise its effects and orient its action and help to obtain more sure and rapid results from the curative point of view.

The traditional homoeopaths are wrong to believe that the strict observation of the law of Similars, without trying to understand it, is always good for the patient. The pathogenesis are really, says Dr. Nebel, some physiopathologic studies of remedies. We should understand the homoeopathic remedies as having physiological actions which may not in practice always give curative results. CANALISATION IS THE ART OF DETERMINING THE ORIENTATION OF THE PHYSIOPATHOLOGICAL ACTION OF THE PRINCIPAL REMEDY BY THE PRESCRIPTION OF THE ONE OR MORE SATELLITE REMEDIES CLEARLY DEFINED.

Now we understand that the rational direction give to Homoeopathic treatment, by observing the law of similars in a really scientific sense, will give to him who will understand its principles, an uncontestable superiority on a too traditional Homoeopathy, practiced without taking into account the Drainage.

Finally I must add, if the readers want a detailed study of the Principles of drainage and canalisation, I will ask them to see Hahnemannian Gleanings, March, 1970. p. 109*

I have included in this book an article on the drainage of the respiratory system. There the readers will find how the remedies are topographically distributed according to their elective actions. The readers will find some more information about drainage in the article. ■■

---

* or what we must not do in Homoeopathy—Jain Publishers.

DISEASE OF THE DIGESTIVE SYSTEM OF THE FIRST INFANCY

We will try in this article to make a brief review of the affections of the digestive apparatus and the troubles of nutrition of children. In order to do that we will have to speak at least in ten chapters about their pathology. But you will see that the number of medicines used for children are very small. We will have to fall back again and again on the same remedies. Among the 7 or 8 columns that we have drawn in our schema we will constantly fall back on *Chamomilla, Belladonna* etc.

We may say that the homoeopathic treatment of children as regards digestive system, is very simple. Here is our plan of study.

1. First of all some generalities from the point of view of constitution and temperament of the child and from the point of view of the general actions of homoeopathic remedies in children.

2. Then we will study the basic remedies which we will describe in detail always indicating the hereditary taints corresponding to the remedies.

3. Then we will give a list of principal remedies that may be prescribed in the digestive troubles and in the nutritional troubles of the infancy.

Constitution & Temperament

Let us consider at first a child at birth. If it is quite natural that if carries with it a cerain heredity and shows more or less some hereditary taints which will not quite apparent during its birth but on the contrary these taints will become apparent as the child will grow. If we consider in the light of general homoeopathic philosophy, the child of the first infancy (*infans*), of the second infancy (*pure*), the adolescent, the adult with their constitutions, their temperaments, we will see that their hereditary taints become evident only lately.

Even at the birth, the child seems to be healthy in general with a life. It will not show any sign of very ancient hereditary syphilis coming from several generations, or tuberculous or other taints only after many years. This is not naturally exact in habitual pathology as regards heredos in whom we immediately detect clear taints, evident stigmas and also in children born of tuberculous patients. These children are sickly and they cannot live if they are not separated from the familial milieu. And this is true as regards the symptoms stamped and more or less recognized by the official school. This will be still more evident when we will study the question of constitution. We may say that the child is born with a vital force which is immense and given during the birth, which will gradually diminish till death or old age.

But if a child has a certain constitution, and if it is possible, during the birth, to foresee what will be its consequences (because it is possible up to a certain point to foresee the diseases from which the child may suffer), which one can do inspite of every thing, only with great prudence because if the constitution, a *Static* is fixed; the temperament, the *Dynamic*, is not fixed. The dynamic behaviour of the patient is completely subject to the vegetative life of the digestive system.

1. The three Osteo-articular Constitution

Let us then consider rapidly the question of Constitution and Temperament.

The constitutions of children are well studied by Dr. A. Nebel. According to him there are three forms of static constitution: *Carbocalcic, Phosphocalcic* and *Fluorocalcic.* He also calls these three constitutions Normo-crinic (*Carbocalcic*), Hypercrinic (*Phosphocalcic*) and Hypocrinic (*Cluorocalcic*) according to the endocrinal troubles that may be associated with them, hyper or hypofunction in a general way.

The indications of constitutions of Dr. A. Nebel is very interesting, but it is necessary that we should consider it with care because though it is certainly true from the clinical point of view, yet it is not experimentally proved.

The descriptions of Dr. A. Nebel as it was given to us in his lecture are, that one can distinguish according to the articulator laxity the *Cluorocalce* whose articulator tissues are very lax; the *Phosphocalcic* has medium laxity of articulator tissues and the *Carbocalcic* has very little laxity. These types correspond to hypophysary troubles.

The three salts of Calcium, specially indicated in children are of the first importance in Homoeopathic therapeutics of children. These three salts help to classify at least clinically the individual patient.

2. Physiological temperament

It is also necessary to consider here the temperament as studied by Dr. Allendy. You know that the occult writers of the middle ages, the traditionalists, studied with Hippocrates the temperaments under the four forms: *Lymphatic, Sanguin, Bilious,* and *Nervous.* These terms may actually no more be used from the physiological point of view. They mean nothing precisely. But Dr. Allendy has explained in his book "Les temperaments" that the above classification may again be taken up on a physiological basis. He has described four types: *Atoniplastic, Toniplastic, Toniaplastic, Toniaplastic, Atoniaplastic.*

He started from the very fecund idea that to understand any organism, it is necessary to take into account the qualitative element on the one hand and the quantitative on the other: The *Tonus* and *Plasticity.*

The child is essentially *Atoni-plastic,* because it has at the same time the tonus and plasticity. It has tonus only in *vitro* we may say. It does not use it always in a rapid and clear way. But on the contrary all the diseases from which it suffers are generalised on the whole organism very rapidly. It has no localising tendency.

The Adolescent (young adult) is *Toni-plastic*, because it has at the same time the tonus and the plasticity which it generalises. It does not localise and fixes very little energy on the lesional plan.

In the Adult age, the individual has still the tonus but he begins to localise. He is therefore *Tomi-aplastic*.

Finally the Old has neither the tonus nor the possibility to generalise. His diseases are more or less fixed in time and space. He is atoni-aplastic.

This classification of Allendy is very interesting and very true as regards children.

If we compare the classification of Allendy with that of Claude Sigaud, *Digestive, Respiratory, Cerebral* and *Muscular*, we may say that the child is before all a predominantly digestive. In the child who has only a vegetative life, the digestive system naturally plays a role of the first importance. From the pathological point of view as well as from the therapeutic point of view the $4/5^{th}$ of the affections of the first infancy are related to nutrition, to digestive system and respiratory system i.e. to say to the two important apparatuses of the vegetative life.

3. The Diet.

Because the child is a digestive type, there is great importance as regard diet. It would be irrational for a homoeopath to try to cure a child of its vomiting, diarrhoea, athrepsia, if the Homoeopathic treatment is not followed by a good revision of physical hygiene and of the diet of the child. The clinic and the hygiene have naturally a step over therapeutics in Homoeopathy as well as in the official treatment. The child is after all a digestive type which can neither walk nor move. The movement, air and sun even, have their place in the question of digestion. Therefore it is necessary when you have to treat child for vomiting or for diarrhoea, that you should begin a good clinic.

4. Rapid and simple action of Homoeopathic remedies

Inspite of this, the role of Homoeopathy, though very frequently adjuvant in benign cases, is however very important for being taken into consideration because it may be the best system of medicine in grave cases. In a child which has digestive troubles of common type, it will be necessary to regularise the diet. When the troubles are serious Homoeopathy steps over diet. The Homoeopathic treatment will then act with some advantages, because the child has no pathological past behind it, because the troubles though serious are not interacted at first as there had not been many diseases that have stepped into one another or succeeded one after the other. There had not been successive morbid metastasis in time and space for which we will not have good results with our Homoeopathic remedies without a thorough search in the antecedents. When we have to treat an adult we are very often forced to find out the chronological succession of the remedies indicated. As for example a woman is of *Natrum muriaticum*, then of *Sepia*, then of *Lachesis* and finally of *Psorinum*. In the case of child we will not have any succession of remedies: there does not exist any pathological past. The child is a new organism. It has come new in the world. Generally we do not find hereditary taints in the child. These taints are there but not *in vitro*. We must investigate the past in the parents, not in the child. And if you add to these facts the idea that the child is extremely sensitive you will easily understand that Homoeopathy has a definite advantage over the chemotherapic treatment of the official school.

5. The part played by the morbid heredity

Thus we arrive at the question of morbid heredity in children which leads us to study at first the Nosodes from the therapeutic point of view.

The little child has therefore an immense vital force, its hereditary taints are shrouded. The famous hereditary Psora of Hahnemann is a term which suits admirably to children. It is at the end of 4, 5, 6, 8 or 10 years and sometimes even later the child will be forced to purge its hereditary taints that it has received. Fortunately its organism will purge them rarely so long as it is a child. The principal means of purge are the eruptive fevers and acute diseases which are special in children: whooping cough, chicken pox, scarlatina, measles etc. The measles is an important infantile disease, which seems to us to be a real collective crisis of the cleansing of entire generation. The measles is an important cleansing disease of tubercular conditions. Scarlatina is related to hereditary psoric, tubercular related to Psorotubercular condition, intricated with sycosis and syphilis. The whooping cough is like measles related to tubercular condition. It is the great antipsorics of Hahnemann that will be able to prevent them, but in this case there will be a spasmodic element which does not exist in case of measles. In the case *Sulphur* will cause rapidly a cutancous eruption. In whooping cough the most important thing is the localized spasm of the larynx. In this case what becomes of the idea of microbe and specific drugs? The microbe exists and it should not be considered negligible. The germs grow because they have a favourable ground and will play, because of its migratory character, the part of sparks the spontaneously spring out of overheated combustibles. In the actual life, and perhaps since thousands of years that man exist, they should necessarily suffer from measles ninety times out of hundred in their childhood. So much so that Psora is so to say, anchored in us in an indefinite manner. Perhaps it had been attracted from the very moment when man began to live in caves or in a house with a roof on it, depriving himself partially of pure open air, of sun and light. Normally when we speak of naturists, about back to the nature, we think of natural food, but none among us will have the idea to live outside like an animal.

But let us not anticipate. What we may say, in reply to the question of heredity—if we admit that its influence does not act only on two or three but on numerous generations – is that the miasms of humanity have fatally left their stamps on the children: *tuberculosis, syphilis, gonorrhoea cancer.* Let us not forget other diseases such as Malaria which was for so long a time of the first importance in our countries as well as in the Orient or in other countries having hot climate.

Those which seem to us more important in our region are:

The *Psora* first of all, i.e. to say chronic tuberculinism of Dr. A. Nebel, probably associated with alimentary intoxications or other.

The *Syphilis* of which the role is well-known, has surely in fluency on numerous generations.

The *Gonorrhoea*, which seems to us very important, though its influence is impossible to prove by the Homoeopathic school that it may hereditarily influence the sycotic temperament in children and in adults. But from multiple facts collected from our experience we are inclined to believe that sycosis plays an important part and it is the cause of different troubles.

Finally malaria and all other possible intoxications by alcohol, meat etc.

For each of these entities we must think of the possibility of human temperamental deviations even though there is no necessity of transmission of grams in children.

The hereditary taints in the child are not evident. They are always veiled. It is only during the second infancy these taints are revealed by means of all sorts of possible affections: eruptive fever, cutaneous troubles, spasmodic troubles and many other diseases that are not possible to enumerate here. ■■

II

The treatment of the troubles of the digestive apparatus and of nutrition of the first infancy.

1. General therapeutic considerations.

How should we treat the child from Homoeopathic point of view when we compare the Homoeopathic treatment of the child with that of the adult? In children we may take into account the question of heredity and use of Nosodes. But precisely because these hereditary taints are more or less dormant, that become evident later on, and precisely because they should reveal themselves very lately, it becomes necessary that we should not treat the child in a brutal manner with Nosodes.

In a general way, we may say that the great antipsorics of Hahnemann, that remedies from plants and minerals are more advantageously used in children than the remedies from the animal kingdom. You will find none of the remedies from animal kingdom on our chart because their actions are very complex. In any case these very rare remedies room the animal kingdom should be used with great care and often in relatively low potency.

As for example we should not treat brutally the child with *Tuberculins* or *Serum of marmoreck,* not because of the chance of aggravation of adult (a child generally tolerates better the Homoeopathic medicines), but because we will not get clear and favourable results. The effects of the great classic remedies are generally favourable. Some Nosodes, *Bacillinum, Medorrhinum Luesinum* may be indicated more often than the habitual tuberculins. On the contrary for a prenatal treatment we may act on the pregnant mother deeply and energetically with all the Nosodes specially by *T. K., T. R. Luesinum.* When the woman is pregnant you may treat her directly for three months for her nausea and vomiting or for her sympathetic troubles. It is only towards the fourth month and up to the end you will treat almost exclusively the child by using alternately *Thuja, Natrum Sulphuricum* on the one hand and *T. R., Medorrhinum* or *Luesinum* on the other hand. This kind of treatment seems to act marvellously as prenatal treatment according to our personal experience.

3

2. Some Rules of Prescription

We are now going to study the most important basic remedies that are used in children. A clinical classification will follow later on which will serve us as the basis of the study of our homoeopathic remedies in different cases.

Let us give at first some rules of prescription for the treatment of children.

We have just said that the child has no pathological past. There is no medicinal aggravation in children. This fact surprises those who come new in Homoeopathy and they are also surprised to see how easy it is to treat the child with homoeopathic medicines. One faces difficulty when one begins to do Homoeopathy with *Sulphur, Lycopodium* and other such remedies that have centrifugal action. These remedies may in some cases cause aggravation of eczema and liver troubles. In children everything goes well. It is generally easy to select a remedy and the organism of the child responds rapidly. It is curious to note that in children the nature seems to be at our disposal. Subjective symptoms are very much necessary in Homoeopathic treatment but in the case of a child and animals it is different. Here the objective symptoms are more important and they are the real keys that will help us to arrive rapidly to the simillimum.

On this question we may automatically make a justified remark to some of the unicists for whom homoeopathy is valuable only in subjective symptoms. They think that the objective symptoms are less important, while some homoeopaths like Dr. A. Nebel have tried to enrich the Homoeopathic pathogenesis with the fruits of their clinical researches with all the indications that one may find on the tongue, on the lips and on the face. These facts have been described but it is a mistake because numerous objective symptoms have been indicated by Hahnemann himself in his pathogenesis specially in case of child.

Rules of Posology

In case of a child use the high dilutions only with care inspite of the fact that the child easily tolerates them because, it is preferable to give the remedies that do not act for a long time. If you apply a very high dilution you will be forced to wait for 3, 4, or 5 months before repeating the medicine according to the general principle of homoeopathy, or you will not be able to use any other remedy and you will not be able to ascertain which of the remedies will have been effective. Or again their action may be very fleeting and you will have the risk to take time. In a child it is necessary to act soon. You should not wait for curing the vomiting of a child or cholera infantile. You should not, like some unicists, turn over the pages of a book for two hours for finding out the good remedy and thus risk the aggravation of the disease. I, however believe that fewer remedies are required for children than for the adult. Generally the cases are simple because there is no pathological past, or if you like the child has his past before it. It is, as it will grow, it will show the signs of hereditary taints in the form of eruptive fevers or other affections. The affections will appear in their time. They should not be called in earlier with a misunderstood treatment, neither they should be "choked" in their appearances by forcing the eruption to get in i.e. suppressed.

A. The Basic Remedies

These are the great antipsorics of Hahnemann of which the list is somewhat revised but on the whole it is exact.

You will be astonished of the following fact: If you consider these remedies you will find that more than half a dozen of these remedies should never be used in children.

Graphites for example is very rarely a remedy of a child. It will begin to be indicated in the 2nd infancy. It is not absolutely a constitutional remedy.

Causticum will be indicated only in the 2nd infancy, in children who have partial paralysis, strabism, or other troubles like retention of urine, incontinence of urine or some manifestations having a peculiar mental symptom: the fear of darkness. But it is not generally in indicated in an infant.

Similarly a child may become a *Thuja* child after vaccination but some time must elapse before the picture, which the British homoeopath Dr. Burnet has so clearly described to us. It is only after vaccination during the second infancy the child may have warts, brittle nails and other symptoms of *Thuja*.

Lachesis, Ignatia, Nux vomica, all these remedies of endocrinal imbalance are also to be considered later on. A girl who in her first infancy will require *Chamomilla* or *Belladonna* will become a patient of *Ignatia* only at puberty. Dr. Nebel sometimes uses *Lachesis* in children before puberty when they are related to *Sulphur.*

Natrum sulphuricum, a remedy of hydrogenoids in particular will be indicated only in the second infancy, in asthmatic children who have the attacks during the second infancy. Asthma of a child is generally amenable to *Phosphorus* and *Natrum muriaticum.*

Many other ground remedies which are suitable to the adolescents, adults or to the second infancy are not indicated in infants.

The remedies of infants are very simple and less numerous.

First of all the three *Calcareous: carbonica, Calcarea phosphorica* and *Calcarea flurica.*

We have said just now that the so fecund and so useful description of Dr. A. Nebel from the clinical point of view of the osteo-articular constitutions should be supported by an experimental basis by quantitative and comparative researches of *Calcium Carbonate, Calcium Phosphate* and *Fluoride of Calcium* in the skeletons of numerous individuals of all ages. We know already that in the bones, there is 2/

3 of *Calcium phosphate* for 20/100 of *Calcium carbonate* and a very small quantity of *Fluoride of calcium.* This fact shows that while the Carbonics are more numerous, the qualitative question is more important than the quantitative in the bone tissues that always contain these three Calcium salts.

Inspite of the above face, it is necessary to make quantitative researches and to have physiological criteria. This is not yet done.

It is also necessary, on the basis of the antagonism of *Silicate* and of *Calcium,* specially *Calcarea carbonica,* to find out what is the quantity of *Silicate* contained in the periarticular tissues because it is said that in the *Fluoro-calcics,* there is a great laxity of the articulations in relation to that laxity if for example there is greater trouble of Silicate metabolism in Fluorocalcics.

Whatever it may be, we may call the age of the infants with Dr. Theories, the age of Calcium and if the child is before all a digestive, we must try to understand how much the question of mineralisation and bones are physiologically and bones are physiologically related to the digestive system.

We see then that from the therapeutical point of view the three *Calcareas* are of the first importance in children. After the Calciums comes *Silicea* and later on *Sulphur* and *Arsenic.*

We therefore find at the basis of Homoeopathic treatment of children, acting as the best of the remedies among the habitual important remedies of morbid temperaments, the minerals that from the human organism and *Arsenic*, which though not a mineral, is at the basis of the constitutions. With them we may add *Phosphorus* but from another point of view it is only of secondary importance.

Really speaking *Phosphorus* has very good action in children of all ages but it is a dangerous remedy because in actual life, most of the children whom we treat are oxyenoid tubercular. they may soon suffer from ganglionary or respiratory lesions and in such cases *Phosphorus* should be used with great care up to the age of 18 to 20. However, there is one exception, in the case of infantile asthma which "responds" to *Phosphorus* 30.

Let us then leave aside *Phosphorus* in case of digestive troubles of children. Let us study at first the five remedies that we have already mentioned. Then we will study *Lycopodium, Sepia, Thuja* and other remedies that are less important: *Natrum muriaticum & Iodium* though they are secondary to those which we have placed on the top of our schema.

Let us first of all study comparatively the three Calcareas: *Calcarea carbonica, Calcarea phosphorica* and *Calcarea fluorica* of which the first two are more important from the clinical point of view.

Calcarea carbonica. It corresponds to all digestive and nutritional troubles of the infants at the beginning of the second infancy. The child suffers from troubles caused by milk which it does not digest. At the end of the 2nd infancy there may be rachitism or some manifestations of nutrition. Nutritional troubles are of the first importance in this remedy. If from the very birth, the child has a big head, protruded frontal eminence, you will immediately think of a heredo-syphilitic child. *Calcarea carbonica* is a very important remedy of some heredo-syphilitic children. It acts also on Fluorocalcis of A. Nebel and *Calcarea carbonica which is considered* as a constitutional remedy of Carbocalicis should not be confounded here. The child cannot digest well the milk and may vomit it in curdled from; it may have acidity, sour stool. It does not like fat and milk with too much fat is not digested by it. *Calcarea carbonica* perfectly suits these children.

Later on in the second infancy *Calcarea carbonica* will evolve towards rachitism and avitaminosis. We will have then the typical child of *Calcarea carbonica:* big, fat, soft, chilly, slow, indolent, always aggravated by cold, who walks late. If it is forced to walk earlier it will become bow-legged and it may have al the troubles or rickets. Thorax becomes shallow, big belly, open fontanelles, perspiration on the head. It suffers from obesity. It becomes a prize-baby. It becomes a prize-baby.

One important characteristic of the child is that it desires indigestible food, chalk, charcoal etc. It seems that the child receives from the nature the indication about his troubles of Calcium metabolism, and it tries to fight against its rachitism by products which are not food. Thus it may have great desire for eggs, salt, sugar, and certain condiments. He may not have appetite.

Silicea. In opposition to *Calcarea carbonica* it is rather a lean child, small with a big head and a big belly. It has also sweat of the head; difficult closing of the fontanelles with early lymphatic ganglions. The ganglions of *Calcarea carbonica* are soft but the ganglions of *Silicea* are hard and small and mobile, rolling under fingers or they may suppurate. The child of *Silicea* may have extraganglionary boils, fistulas, coetaneous boils, respiratory boils and chronic otitis etc.

Silicea has also sour erutations like *Calcarea carbonica*. The child may have diarrhoea but more often constipation. It has troubles after vaccination. Very often the child who will be suitable to *Thuja* and will have warts towards the age of 10, will require at first *Silicea*.

Silicea is a remedy of the troubles of growth and athrepsia. *Calcarea carbonica* suits rather to rickets. *Silicea* may grow to become lean; *Calcarea carbonica* will grow towards obesity.

Calcarea phosphorica has retracted boat like chest, the opposite of *Calcarea carbonica*. *Calcarea phosphorica* child will suffer often from colic with every trail with new food. It has diarrhoea from fruits, from fruit juices. *Calcarea phosphorica* is tubercular and chronic tubercular which cause in it a desire for exciting foods, either alcohol or meat. *Calcarea phas* phorica has rather the desire for porks, and salted meat. It is a remedy of Phosphocalcic child, either pure or mixed with marked hereditary tubercular condition.

In *Calcarea phosphorica*, like *Calcarea carbonica* and *Silicea* the fontanelles close late and the child evolves towards anaemia of the muscles. Its tissues are soft. Really speaking *Calcarea phosphorica* is not a remedy of rickets.

Calcarea fluorica. In *Calcarea fluorica* there exists a great laxity of articulations. The articulations are very lax but the glands are very hard, as hard as stones. The bad elastic tissues are seen on the surface of the veins. The child will have varicose veins in adult age. The rachitism of *Calcarea fluorica* is related to Syphilitic heredity (with deformations of bones like curvature of the femur, of the tibia etc.). Heredo-syphilis is marked specially on the sense organs. The child will have in the very early age, suppurations of the eye lids, blepharitis, otitis etc.

Some Homoeopaths use Luesinum as a rule with *Calcarea fluorica* and *Aurum metallicum* specially in children who suffer from otitis and during dentition. Teething is particularly difficult in *Calcarea fluorica* because the child has not enough place in his maxilla, so that the teeth may grow easily. The teeth grow obliquely. You may see all the signs of syphilitic heredity on the teeth, for example dented teeth, the ogival palate etc. *Calcarea fluorica* corresponds to this picture.

After these four very important constitutional remedies are to be studied. We will speak at first of *Iodium* and *Natrum muriaticum*. They will be required somewhat late, generally at the end of the first infancy or during the second infancy.

Natrum muriaticum. It is a remedy of the troubles of growth of children who remain lean for a longtime, who do not develop well or who remain a cretin.

As regards cretinism, the child who is very slow to develop is also suitable to *Silicea,* to *Natrum Muriaticum* or specially to *Baryta crbonica.* In such cases we should think of a very ancient syphilis which has attacked the endocrines specially the hypophisary. *Baryta carbonica* will be the specific remedy of heredo-syphilitic, *Silicea* of the heredo-tubercular and *Natrum muriaticum* 200 being the constitutional remedy for fixing the salts of Calcium and to help the child to gain weight.

We must compare *Natrum muriaticum* with *Serum de Quinton* or with *Aqua Marina*. In some patients lower triturations of *Natrum muriaticum* are necessary. It is Arnulphy, a famous homoeopath of Nice, who first proved the value of this remedy. Arnulphy worked with Quinton.

Our colleague Jarricot of Lyon continued the use of *Serum de Quinton*. Unfortunately, I believe that actually this remedy is very rarely used. However, it is a valuable arm in many cases of athrepsia or of nutritional troubles of the infants.

Iodium. It is to be given in cases of marasmus or to children suffering from indurated glands with troubles of nutrition. The child eats well but becomes lean and evolves rapidly towards tuberculosis. But this remedy is more interesting in the second infancy.

Thuja. It is equally useful in the 2nd infancy for troubles relating to sycosis and vaccination.

Sulphur. A child may soon require *Sulphur. Sulphur* is generally called the king of antipsorics. For Hahnemann *Caicarea carbonica* was the king of Antipsorics. He considered the value of heredity because the more one is a Homoeopath the more he gives importance to heredity from the pathological and therapeutic point of view. We shall not hesitate to go or three generations only as some homoeopaths teach. But *Sulphur* has as well as *Calcarea carbonica*, a deep action on hereditary taints.

In the symptoms that indicate the primordial agent of hereditary force in *Calcarea carbonica*, we should note one very important symptom, the mydrasis. It is a child suitable to *Calcarea carbonica*. In acute case *Chamomilla* or *Belladonna* is necessary.

Sulphur will therefore be necessary to drain out, in a brutal manner, all the possible toxins. It is with *Sulphur* we will begin the treatment of measles, whooping cough and most of the infantile diseases.

Sulphur is inconvenient only, as explained by P. Chavanon, in children who have easy supportive tendency. We will help the nature of play the part of fire, and the condition of the child will ameliorate at the cost of a possible otitis or any other suppuration that may become dangerous. A single dose of *Sulphur* given prematurely to a child who has the maximum suppurative tendency, will improve the general condition, but will aggravate the local conditions. There is therefore antagonism between general and local interest of the organism.

Sulphur is an important remedy and should be used in lower or medium dilutions and should be very rarely repeated.

The important indications of *Sulphur*, though it does not enter in the present study, is the incontinence of urine. With *Calcarea carbonica*, *Sulphur* is of the first importance in incontinence of urine in children. It is with *Sulphur* 200 followed by *Plantago* 6 and *Equisitum* 30 we will have frequent and regular success in the treatment of bed wetting in children.

Besides will find cramp rings almost always in the iris of these children and hereditary syphilis.

Lycopodium. It is a remedy of children of all ages.

I have *Lycopodium* in our scheme immediately after *Calcarea* and *Sulphur* because there are digestive troubles which are related either to cutaneous sphere (*Sulphur*) or to the liver (*Lycopodium*).

The principal indication of *Lycopodium* is loss of appetite in all ages.

There is hardly a child in whom we cannot bring back the appetite. I have never failed even in a single case. Anorexia called nervous or mental seems to us in reality to be of hepatic origin because we cure it by liver remedies. It is here, where homoeopathy is really interesting because here we have to make a particular mental gymnastic. The officials at first make a pathogenesis and they gather a group of symptoms. The difficulty is that there is often a great distance between diagnosis and therapeutics. There is often an abyss to cross. One may not always cross over this difficulty. In homoeopathy we have always some landmark in our reasoning. From symptoms to therapeutics, from therapeutics to clinic our mind shuttles many times and we have constantly the confirmation by touch-stone treatment. We may bring back the appetite of infants or of children of the 2nd infancy or of girls at the time of puberty who keep themselves closed in a room, who like solitude. Their condition is cured with *Sepia.* When puberty will make them hypertensive of the portal veins and when there is pelvic and liver congestion, we will be bring back their appetite. We will cure the mental type of anorexia of the first or of the second infancy. We therefore think that we are right to think that if every time we cure them with remedies like *Lycopodium* or by other remedies of hepatic insufficiency, that the anorexia which is called mental is in reality of hepatic origin or perhaps hepatopancretic origin. It may exist with some mental troubles, but it is before all glandular and is often related to more or less ancient hereditary syphilis.

We will cure marvelously some nervous anorexias with *Lycopodium* in children who are soon satisfied, who leave always half of their milk.

Lycopodium will also be useful in cyclic vomiting with Senna.

B. Functional remedies of different syndromes of nutrition.

Now we come to the properly called homoeopathic remedies. Let us examine some syndromes of nutrition from the clinical point of view.

1. Athrepsia, congenital weakness, anaemia.

2. Troubles of growth, rickets and its satellite troubles

3. All the liver troubles with *Lycopodium,* from mental anorexia to acetonomy.

4. Vomiting, diarrhoea, dyspepsia, infantile cholera, dys-

entery, enterocolitis and constipation, are the most important syndromes. Then we will broach rapidly colics, constipations and we will say something on erythema which is related to digestive troubles.

1. Athrepsia, congenital weakness, anaemia.

These diseases are classic in children who are brought up with artificial milk or with food that does not contain sufficient vitamins. We have no homoeopathic remedy like fruit vitamins and we will also give orange juice or juices of other fruits. We will however follow the principles of naturists and will give one or two drops daily while the official school will apply quantity of acid fruit juice daily. We will thus avoid the troubles of demineralisation.

But when we have children suffering from marasmus, who are mere skeletons without flesh and who rapidly proceeds towards death we will think of *Silicea* (30 or even 200); *Natrum muriaticum, Iodium,* the basic remedies and in the Materia Medica we will find some more important remedies: *Abrotanum, Arsenicum iodatum,* iodatum, which are very important in pre-tubercular or tubercular children who become emaciated very rapidly. They should be used in the 3rd dilution or in triturations. In other cases *Calcarea silicate* in chilly children. *Ferum metallicum* and *Pulsatilla* will be indicated in anemic children (anaemia of children for want of air). In such cases quantity of milk should be diminished and food with assimilable iron should be used.

In such cases we may use *Ferum metallicum* 30. *Pulsatilla* is an excellent drainer of tubercular patients. Children suffering from marasmus are more or less tubercular.

2. Rickets, troubles of growth.

In rickets we have spoken of *Calcarea carbonica, Silicea, Lycopidium*, afterwards *Natrum muriaticum* & *Abrotanum*. We should also think of *Baryta carbonica* which is the best remedy of cretinism of children who cannot speak well, who walk late, who are intellectually late. *Baryta carbonica* is one of the principal remedies in retarded children. We should also think of *Luesimum* and *Hepato-Luesinum*. The latter seems very often more active.

Sulphur iodatum may indicated in emaciation of children, in oxygenoid children of tubercular constitution. Dr. Parteneau has given a prescription having a reconstituting power which is very useful in children. Here is the formula.

Sulphur 6
Iodium 6
Calcarea Phos ⎫
Calcarea carb ⎬ IX
Calcarea flour ⎭

It is good medicinal combination which will help the emaciated child to take up weight. It seems that the lower dilutions of *Iodium* and *Sulphur* are necessary and *Natrum muriaticum 200* will also be necessary to fix the salts of

Calcium.

Oleum jecoris aselli (codliver oild), may be given in homoeopathy. When it is too much diluted, I believe, does not act. It may be given according to the official doses, but it may cause digestive troubles.

Thus we come to the question of Vitamins.

We should also think of Organotherapy in all cases of the troubles of growth. We must not forget that syphilis is the basic factor of endocrinal troubles, next comes tuberculosis.

In children of tubercular constitution *Arsenicum iodatum* helps the child to take up weight and *Kali iodatum* in syphilitic child.

Aurum metallicum may be added to the list.

3. Anorexia and hepatic troubles

In *Anorexia* the important basic remedy is *Lycopodium* but it should often be followed by remedies directly acting on nausea and vomiting such as *Ipecac* and *Antimonium crudum,* according as the tongue is clean or covered with white patch.

In anorexia of children I generally give *Lycopodium* 30 one dose every 10 days, *Calcarea phos* 6, sometimes *Arsenicum album* and sometimes *Silcea* according to the symptoms.

If there is vomiting *Ipecac* is indicated.

When there is acetonemic vomiting Belladonna, Senna, Causticum, Lycopodium.

In these cases *Lecithin* may be given in gross doses. *Lecithin* has sometimes good actions.

On the whole with a few remedies *Anorexia* may be cured.

Sepia may be given in the second infancy when the child eats and digests only what is defended to it. Hard cheese, vinaigre, salted food (like *Phosphorus* & *Natrum muriaticum*) *Sepia* will be indicated in children of *Iodium* type who desires to remain alone.

Really speaking *Sepia* is remedy of *Anorexia* of girls of 14, 15 or 16 years of ages, who have arrived at the age of puberty, who isolate themselves and say eating is a taxation to them. We can cure them easily with *Sepia* 200 & *Nux vomica* 30 followed by *Luesinum*. If the cure is delayed *Luesinum* should be used alternately with *Lycopodium*.
(SYPHILINUM)

4. Vomiting and Diarrhoea

In vomiting and diarrhoea I will place *Aethusa cynapium* on the top of the list. But Dr. Renard has convinced me about the great value of *Ipecac* in infants. Let Dr. Renard speak.

Dr. Renard—*Ipecac* is indicated not only in the vomiting

of infants but also in diarrhoea of infants. There are children who have alternate diarrhoea and constipation. The stools may be green; the colour of the stool may be normal when passed but becomes green afterwards. *Ipecac* should be given not in dilution but in mother tincture, one drop with hot water, sometimes 2 drops a dose four times a day.

Dr Bernoville—We may then say that it is a marvellous remedy but it should be used in the required doses.

Generally when you have to treat mechanical troubles i.e. materially palpable troubles such as digestive troubles, lower dilutions even the mother tincture should be used. For sympathetic troubles and mental troubles and mental troubles the high dilutions are required as for example you may use *Ipecac* 30 or 200 in asthma. If you want to cure the fit of whooping-cough use *Ipecac* 6 or 30.

Aethusa cynapium—*Aethusa cynapium* and *Antimonium crudum* are also two interesting remedies. The second is to be given in vomiting of children having a white washed tongue, and temperament like that of a *Calcarea carbonica* child.

Aethusa cymapium is a very important remedy. It is remedy of the Ombellifera family and like all other remedies of this family it has spasms with all its troubles; sudden vomiting immediately after sucking or taking milk; vomiting of big clots of milk. It is a very faithful remedy. Generally it is given in the 6th dilution.

You see that generally the homoeopathic therapeutics is easy in children. The remedies are less numerous and easy to handle.

In cyclic vomiting *Iris versicolor, Mercurius dulcis,* and *Senna* give good results. The vomiting may be acetonemic when *Senna* will give good result.

In diarrhoea there are many remedies easy to handle. These remedies are of vegetable and mineral origin. The minerals seem to act slowly but deeply while the vegetable act very rapidly specially in acute cases.

In infantile cholera we should chose from among *Veratrum album, Antimonium crudum, Cuprum,* and *Camphora.*

Veratrum and *Camphora* are more imporltant in infantile cholera where there is the danger of collapse of the heart; the child becomes ice-cold, cyanotic, having cold sweat on the forehead during and after stool.

Camphora has the pinched nose, the face is cold. The stage of collapse.

I repeat again here *Veratrum* is more important, then comes *Cuprum* and *Comphara. Antimonium crudum* is indicated in more benign cases.

These remedies are also of the first importance in Asiatic cholera. In France this disease is now absent. Homoeopathy has taken its root in countries where there is an epidemic of this terrible disease. In Brazil, Homoeopathy has obtained the official consideration since the epidemic of yellow fever in which Homoeopathy was so much successful that it is recognised by the official authorities.

These remedies act in infantile cholera as well as in Asiatic cholera.

Chamomilla, Podophyllum and *China* may be compared and all the three act well when the stool is clear yellow.

Chamomilla has the stool like that of rotten egg mixed as if with chopped spinach. Diarrhoea during dentition like that of *Podophyllum,* specially indicated in diarrhoea in the summer or during hot climate. The child has tendency to prolapsus of the anus.

China is to be used when there is great dehydration with diarrhoea.

Mercurius solubilis and *Mercurius corrosivus* have greenish stools but those of the first is mixed with mucous, aggravation during night. The mouth of the patients is humid with thirst, the tongue is swollen, having imprint of the teeth.

Mercurius corrosives has stomatitis and tenasmus of the abdomen or of the rectum. There may be ulceration and terrible pains.

Agentum nitricum, Ipecac and *Aconite* have green stools.

Ipecac has stools like chopped spinach.

Aconite is an excellent remedy when the child has green stools with agitation, anxiety and great thirst.

Argentum nitricum has also greenish stools. Abuse of sweets. Stools become green rapidly. Stools, immediately after suckling.

Ipecac has green stools, sometimes glairy, sometimes mixed with blood. Cramping pain around the naval region.

Belladonna may also be indicated in green stools with spasmodic constriction of the anus. The important character is aggravation by the least contact. The child does not like that one touches his belly.

Magnesia carbonica and *Rheum*, with *Calcarea carbonica* are the three remedies of sour smelling stool in children.

Aethusa. We have already studied this remedy.

Kreosotum is indicated in children who have dental troubles. Caries of teeth which become black and crumbles.

Kali bichromickum is to be compared with *Mercurius solubilis* and specially in dysentery (*Ipecac, Kali bichromicum, Arsenicum, Mercurius corrosives,* are specially used in bacillary dysentery).

Capsicum is useful in muco-membranous entrocolitis, with much burning sensation, false membranes in stools.

Solics. In *colics of* infants *Chamomilla* is the remedy of angry children who should be always carried, who have dental troubles like that of *Belladonna* and *Mercurius solubilis*.

Belladonna has fever and throbbing pains; *Chamomilla* is irritable and capricious; *Mercurius solubilis* has aggravation at night and in the heat of the bed.

China has diarrhoea with much flatus in the abdomen.

Colocynth has amelioration by doubling forward or by drawing the legs on the abdomen.

Veratrum album has great abdominal pain; infantile cholera.

Magnesia phosphorica has the same modality like that of *Colocynth*.

Dioscorea also is to be thought of (when there is amelioration by bending backwards).

Constipation: In constipation the remedies are very easy to apply. We will apply *Calcarea, Lycopodium, Natrum muriaticum* followed by *Bryonia* and *Taraxacum*, two very Important remedies.

Bryonia when the child has no desire of stools. When the stools are brown and large in quantity.

Taraxacum when the constipation is of hepatic origin. It acts better in 3x. It has map-like tongue. *Natrum muriaticum* has also somewhat similar tongue.

Graphitis is interesting in fat children having tendency to obesity and chilliness.

Opium is interesting in constipation without desire. It is to be given in the 30ᵗʰ potency like *Bryonia*. Stools are hard and like small balls.

Magnesia muriaticum is a related to *Natrum muriaticum* as regards dry stools, which comes out in crumbs.

Alumina is a remedy of constipation without desire. The patient is constipated even when the stools are soft. It is also useful in coetaneous troubles and erythema.

Coetaneous troubles and erythema. *Chmomilla* and *Belladonna* are useful in erythema with extreme hypersensitive skin specially during dentition. In *Belladonna* there is the classic trade; *redness, heat and pain.*

Rhus toxicodendron and *Causticum* should be given if there are vesicles (small vesicles *Rhus tox,* large vesicles *Causticum*). In pemphigus *Rhus toxicodendron* and *Causticum* may be useful.

When there is hereditary taints *Luesimum* or *Hepato-Luesimum* and sometimes *Lycopodium* or other ground remedies are to be used.

In cases of traumatism or reddish skin aggravated or caused by: too much tight dresses *Arnica* is to be used.

We should also treat local infections by external application *Calendula* or *Calendula* ointment, or drying power such as talcum.

HOMOEOPATHY IN ACUTE INFANTILE DISEASES OF THE RESPIRATORY SYSTEM

It is not our intention to give a complete treatment of the diseases of the respiratory system of the first and the second infancy in this article, but it will not be wanting in utility and interest. We have willingly restricted ourselves in giving some general ideas about the facts that we have observed during our practice while treating children with homoeopathic medicines and to add the pathogenic study of remedies of which the indications are more frequent in course of respiratory diseases of children.

Our experience is enough to say that in infantile pathology, more than that of the adult and the old, Homoeopathy compared with Allopathy, has been proved to be the treatment of choice either it is considered from the angle of doctrinal conceptions or it is considered from pragmatic aspect of therapeutic results. It is besides in the treatment of children every Allopath crosses the threshold of a somewhat mysterious homoeopathy and voluntarily desists himself from the audacity of assuming the treatment of an acute case with imponderable doses absolving himself at the bottom of his heart of the excuse "that the infantile pharmoacopea of Allopathy is extremely limited and that the useful dose is so near to the toxic dose that one is right to be afraid of,"

We therefore admit of that fear which is human, and is the beginning of wisdom and that the dose in medicine in the treatment of children becomes a possibility in favour of homoeopathy. When, after some good results, the new doctor has gained some confidence on his method and when he timidly extends it to **adult and to old, he soon finds that it is in children** his method is specially success-ful.

In fact it is a truism that the children are eminently sensitive to our dilutions for some proved or hypothetical reasons that we have not discussed here. It is thus the method takes form. On the one hand it is inoffensive and fecund and on the other hand, so far as we concerned, we believe that the theories of Hahnemann, applied to the diseases of the first infancy offer another source of interest.

The facts that we have witnessed, have convinced us to recognise the exactitude and importance of the notions of morbid ground, of constitutions, of temperaments, of he-reditary pathological predispositions. There is no doubt that we are not in a position to prove them with laboratory arguments, but the concrete reality concords exactly with the theories so that one has the right to accept them with a favourable presumption.

We are particularly interested here in acute pneumopathies of infants, and here is in summary some of the deductions that we believe to be true.

The acute diseases of the respiratory tract of children do not come as a bolt from the blue or as if the organism is suddenly succumbed under the attack of brutal microbes. Before the appearance of the disease the child possesses within it some possibilities of diseases.

What are these preparing possibilities? First of all the ground, specially tubercular. We have worked in a region where no familial heredity was unknown to us and our field of action was vast enough to give us numerous opportunities to make comparisons. The more a family stock is encumbered with tuberculosis, the more there are the risks of an acute affection of the respiratory system in lower ages in the descendants, particularly broncho-pneumonia. The prognosis itself will be as much grave as the familial taint is more charged.

Besides the ground, there is the second factor which is very important for the preparation of the ground. It is the chill. It is customary to read in the medical treatises, that the chill is an "occasional" physical cause. But we add that "it is the opportunity that makes the thief."

The part played by the chill in acute pneumopathies is considerably important. Its causes are different. It may be imputable to bad hygiene, insufficiently heated room, exposition to air current, negligence of the parents who let go out their children insufficiently guarded or dressed. These children generally already suffer from cold. In other cases the catching of cold may be of more general nature such as the consequence of sudden variation of atmospheric temperature or a prolonged coldness. The cause of pneumonia, bronchopneumonia, pulmonary congestions and corticopleuritis by the first heat, or when the days are hot and nights are cold. We think that the ground and the chill are absolutely important and during our last years of practice, we were in the habit of advising preventive measures to our clients, recommending them to keep their children, who are suffering from cold, hot and sufficiently dressed specially when the atmospheric condition is not favourable and when we doubt the power of resistance of the child.

As regards secondary pneumopathies, the interpretation of the origin is less different. The ground and the chill play no less an important cause. It is specially in children having tubercular constitution you will have the fear of complications: otitis, mastoiditis pleuropneumonia, pleuresy etc. But there is an other cause of complications which we have frequently observed. it is intempstive allopathic treatment. We could have cited numerous cases. We will relate here two cases which are striking.

A girl of 4 years old, having perfect resistance, is attacked since 24 hours, with measles with generalised exanthema appeared in the best of conditions. Cough and . trachitis; temp. 40^0 Symptoms are ordinary, nothing serious. The attending physician under the pretext of avoiding complications and to lower down the temperature gave an injection of vaccine. Four hours after the eruptions retro-ceded, the fever began to osciliate irregularly, marasmus set in and the child died within two hours.

A baby of 9 months, breast fed, having a very good health, has since 24 hours all the general stethoscopic symptoms of bronchopneumonia. His doctor gave towards I 'o' clock in the morning a vaccine. The condition became serious. I was called for consultation. I found complete blockage of the lungs, symptoms of meningitis and a temperature of 40°. I gave a homoeopathic prescription but the child died before the administration of the medicine.

Dr. Allendy has shown with demonstrative arguments that when one opposes the natural course of the disease, there is caused a morbid transfer or metastasis as well as the inhibition of the organism which may lead to worst catastroph. The complications are infinitely rare in children if they are homeopathically treated. In pneumopathies we have been able to cause complete disappearance in our patients the para or metapnemonic abcess as well as purulent pleuresy.

Now, what is the role of microbe and of contagion in the affections? According to us the virulency of the microbes become real only when there is the preparing causes that we have described. As regards contagion, except whooping cough, we do not attach to it any real value.

In summary we may say that homoeopathy is doubly

fecund in these affections. Thanks to the ideas about the ground and atmospheric etiologic factor it may act preventively and avoid the disease. Having said this we may also say that Homoeopathy is non-toxic, and when judiciously applied in the individual case, it has the maximum chance to cure. Finally Homoeopathy is in a favourable position to formulate a prognosis.

After these preliminaries we are going to pass in review a number of remedies among those which are more frequently indicated in the acute diseases of the respiratory system of children. Our study will not be complete. We have tried to bring together the symptoms, to evaluate precisely the indications of each remedy, and we hope that it is done in such a manner that the formulation will be useful to practitioners.

The remedies of the acute affections

Aconite—Affection caused by **dry cold weather,** acute, sudden appearance of the disease. High fever. Thirst for cold water. Hot and dry skin. Extreme agitation with anxiety. Rapid, hard, tense pulse which cannot be depressed. Violent dry cough. Plethoric child, having good constitution, **more sanguin than nervous.**

Used at the beginning of **coryza adenoiditis,** bronchitis, pneumonia and broncho-pneumonia. Stridulus larynigitis.

Allium cepa—Sneezing aggravated in the heat, amelioration in open air. **Watery nasal flow,** corrosive, abundant with irritation of the nostrils. Intense non-irritating lachyrmation **photophobia.** Coryza of infants, causing difficulty of sucking. His fever.

Ammonium carbonicum—Obstruction of the nose, aggravated at night. **Obstruction of the nose of the infants.** Sleeps with open mouth. Cough with rales of mucous, cannot expectorate. Dyspnoea with **intense weakness.** Weak heart. Synocope. Aggravation towards 3o'clock in the morning. Affections of the respiratory system involving the bronchili. Syncopal tendency.

Antimonium tartaricum. Bronchili and alveoles are full of mucous which the patient cannot expectorate. Danger of being asphyxiated. Auscultation reveals all sorts of rales. Pale skin, cynosis of the extremities. Rapid, small pulse. Thirst for cold water, **nausea.** Child weeps when one approaches it. Need for fresh air. Fanning of nostrils. Somnolence, drowsiness. Its place is after *Ipecac* when *Ipecac* not have the desired effect. At this stage, cough becomes less frequent, expectoration dimineshes. An important remedy of capillary bronchitis or bronchopneumonia where it gives unexpected good results.

Apis melifica—A remedy of oedema and exudation. Indicated in the oedema of glottis with amelioration by cold drinks. Meningitis with influenza or acute pneumopathy. Acute piercing cry during sleep. Delirium, stupor, leading to coma. Pain in the head where the child puts its hands. The child rolls its head. The head falls below the pillow. It throws away its covers. Tries to keep itself away from any source of heat. Ameliorations by cold compress. It is indicated for hastening the resorption of pleural exudation.

Arsenicum album—Watery coryza, less abundant, very **excoriating** with irration of the nostrils and upper lip. Amelioration by the application of heat. Cough with frothy expectoration. The patient must sit up for respiration. It cannot lie stretched. Dry lips, the tongue as if roasted, covered with sticky and Foetid mucous. Burning in the pharynx which is dry and red. Great thirst of small quantity of cold water frequently. Extreme weakness with agitation. Aggravation towards 1 A. M. Burning pains in the thorax, upper part of the light lung and pharynx. Trachitis, influenza, pneumonia, bronchopneumonia. The case is always grave and a dynamic. May be given from the very first day of the attack in the 30th dilution once a day specially when clinically the disease is alarming. Influenza, acute pneumopathy.

Arsenicum iodatum—A very important remedy of convalescence from disease of the respiratory system of children of tubercular constitution. The child is vivacious, irritable and impatun. Aggravation in extreme temperatures. Amelioration in open air. Adenopathies. Pneumonia having the tendency to become choronic. Asthma, convalescence, pretubercular condition.

Arum triphyllum—A remedy characterised by irritation

and dryness of the mucous membranes. Excoriation of the lips and of the nostrils with great desire to scratch. The child picks it squamus upper lip which causes burning and inflammation. Ulceration of the nostrils and of the lips. Foetid ulcerating salivation. Deep red mucous membranes of the mouth. Difficult deglutition. Nervous break down. Aggravation in the heat. A right-sided remedy. Infantile diseases of grave a dynamic type. Laryngitis. Aphonia after *over work*.

Baptisia—Grave infectious conditions of **typhoid type.** May be indicated in acute pulmonary affections with prostration, pains of the muscles and bruised feeling. The side on which the patient lies down becomes painful. Delirium. Believes that his extremities are separated from the body. Foetied breath and foetidness of all excretion. Parrot tongue. Influenza, bronchopneumonia, pneumonia.

Belladonna-With *Aconite* and *Ferrum phos,* it form the trio of remedies of the onset of acute diseases. **Sudden onset,** during cold weather (dry or humid).Symptoms appear suddenly. Extreme agitation alternating with prostration. Redness and paleness of the face with sweats. Thirst. Rapid, full tense pulse but **can be depressed.** Suits better to nervous children (remedy of students). *Aconite* being the remedy of villagers). Aggravation by movements (contrary-*Aconite*). Amelioration by cold application and in warm room. Acute delirium with prostration. Dryness of the nostrils and of the larynx with suffocating spasms. Dry, short laryngial cough, at night with painful points in the chest.

Indicated in all acute diseases of the respiratory system at the onset, in false croup, in meningitis, congestion of the brain, convulsions. **At the beginning of all the diseases of the respiratory system.**

Bronium-**Sudden inflammation of the respiratory** tract after a chill (sweat, current of air) when the weather is very hot, in children who are very hotly clothed during the first heat of May or June or during humid weather. Excoriating nasal flow with obstruction of the nose, first the right nostril then extending to the left. Spasmodic dry cough with expectoration. Sensation of *Sulphur* fumes in the bronchili. Laryngo-trachal rales with difficult inspiration. Rapid formation of false membranes. Tendency to adenitis. **Amelioration on the sea side** and by movement, aggravation while eating and drinking (cold drinks), from the evening till the midnight, while entering in a room (cough)—Acute coryza, false croup, laryngotrachitis, bronchitis.

Bryonia-An important remedy of the respiratory system Chronologically its place is just after *Aconite, Belladonna* and *Ferrum phos.* Dryness of the mucous membranes. Intense thirst of large quantity of cold water at long intervals. Dry coryoza with frontal headaches (suppressed catarrhal headaches). Dry cough with tickling of the larynx, aggravation **while entering in a hot room,** with painful points in the chest at fixed points (mobile points –*Kali carb*) specially on the right side. Sticky, brick-red expectoration. Abundant hot sweat causing amelioration. Coryza, **trachitis,**

bronchitis, pneumonia, **bronchopneumonia** where it may be used in period when the disease is fully developed. **Pleuresy.**

Camphora-A very important remedy of sudden chill. If it is applied in time it can check croyza, bronchitis, even acute pneumopathies. It should be taken at the very sensation of chill, at the time of shivering or when "one feels that has caught cold", before the stage of sneezing. If one is sensitive to cold one should keep this remedy in his pocket. Coryza with stopped nose, pain in the head. Aggravation by cold but **does not like to be covered.** Amelioration by heat by hot drinks. Excellent remedy of collapse stage. Weakness and chill being the dominant characteristics (Sweat-*Veratrum album*) Coryza, pneumonia, broncho-pneumonia, capillary bronchitis.

Cantharis—It is specially a remedy of pleuresy. According to Dr. Charge it should be given exactly when the fever begins to decrease, the pain has diminished and disappeared. Exudation continues to increase or persist. The pulse is small, frequent. Humid skin; sweat. Frequent cough. Oliguria.

Causticum—**Hoarseness in the morning.** Sensation of ulcer in the Larynx. Dry expiratory cough, amelioration by drinking cold water. A version to sugar. Nervous and timid child having extreme fright of darkness. Aggravation during clear and beautiful weather, in dry cold wind. Amelioration during rainy or wet season, by hot air Laryngitis, bronchitis.

Carbo vegetabilis—In children, it is a remedy of **grave agonising stage.** Its place comes when *Arsenic* and *Antim. tart.* have failed and the disease goes on increasing towards death. Extreme weakness (*Arsenic, Muriatic acid*). Collapse stage, moribund. Cold breathing. Skin cold with cyanosis, sweat, involuntary Foetid stools. Superficial rapid respiration; **need for fresh air,** wants to be fanned. Small, uncountable rapid pulse. Thready pulse. The condition seems hopeless. *Carbo vegetabilis* given in such a condition often cause resurrection.

Corallia—A remedy of whooping-cough-like cough. Violent spasmodic cough in rapid succession which causes the child to lose its breath. It becomes red, light violent. Complete break-down after the attack. Great weakness. Aggravation in the morning.

Coccus Cacti—Violent cough with viscous mucous. Thready mucous which hangs from the lower lip. Better after expectoration. Spasmodic cough in the morning. Tickling in the larynx. Vomiting of mucous ends the cough. Better while walking. Aggravation while lying on the left side, after sleep, by touch. Whooping cough, trachitis.

Cuprum metallicum—Spasmodic cough with possible convulsion. Amelioration by drinking cold water. Contraction of the extremities (closed fists). Face first red then violet. **A very important remedy of whooping cough.** In case of failure give *Cuprum Aceticum.*

Dulcamara—Stopped nose and cough after exposition to humid cold or during a sudden change of hot weather into cold and humid. It is specially a remedy of affections caused by humid cold, while *Aconite* is a remedy of affections caused by dry cold. **Amelioration by inspiration of hot air.** Aggravation by cold air. Intense thirst for cold water. Rhino-pharyngitis, bronchitis, influenza.

Drosera—Inflammation of the laryngial mucous mem-branes with tickling of the pharynx and larynx. Dry spas-modic cough like the crowing of a cock. Repeated attack of cough with fear of suffocation. The face of the child becomes red, violet, seems swollen. Expectoration of mucous with streaks of blood or vomiting. Expectoration and vomiting ameliorate. During attack the child catches hold of its throat or places its hand on the painful parts. It agitates because movement gives it relief. Better immediately when the child lies down at night and after mid-night. Often epistaxis, constipation. Whooping cough or whooping-cough like cough. Laryngitis, laryngotrachitis, or bronchitis. Whooping cough.

Eupatorium—Influenza with bruised feeling, with great muscular and bone pains. Pain in the chest. Extreme sensi-tiveness to cold. Movement does not ameliorate. Fever with chill and shivering. **Bone pains** with chill. Thirst before chill, the sweat. Sadness and complete breakdown. Dry cough which jerks the patient painfully. Loss of voice in the morning. Influenza, pneumonia, bronchopneumonia, capillary bronchitis.

Euphrasis—An important remedy of Coryza. Abundant mucous discharge with lachrymation. Nasal discharge is not excoriating while the discharge from the eyes is excoriating and acrid (opposite, **All cep.**) Aggravation in the bed, in a **hot room,** in the evening, by humidity and in open air. Coryza, rhinophyaryngitis, conjunctivitis

Ferrum Phosphoricum—Very important in the treatment of children. It should be known well clinically. It has its place between *Aconite* and *Belladonna* when the differentiation between the two does not seem very clear. Less nervous than *Belladonna*. Less plethoric than *Aconite*. *Aconite, Belladonna* and *Ferrum Phos,* are the trio that are used in fever of the infancy. They should also be thought of when from the onset the **disease seems serious.** Non-resistant child. Easily prostrated, **soft pulse,** rapid, easily becomes irregular. Congestive heat with alternating red and pale face. Aggravation in the second part of the night, by movement, by noise, by cough. Amelioration by cold application. It is indicated at the beginning of all fevers on the clinical symptoms: adenoiditis, otitis, rhinopharyngitis, bronchitis, pneumonia, bronchopneumonia, capillary bronchitis.

Glesemium—Tendency to cold, to influenza by humid heat, when hot season changes into cold. Sensation of fullness, obstruction at the base of the nose, often one-sided, specially the left one. Photophobia. Fever with shivering and **need for being covered hotly.** Rhinopha ryngitis, trachitis; heaviness of the limbs, slow pulse, absence of thirst, desire to remain alone.

Hepar Sulphur—The least cold cause Coryza, with obstruction of the nose. Aggravation by cold air. Loss of voice, worse in the morning.

Hard barking cough, **very much aggravated by cold,** by uncovering, in the bed, by putting out the hands from under the covers. Easy sweat, specially at night, which does not cause amelioration. At the end of respiratory diseases or in chronic case *Hepar Sulphur* is characterised by **thick acrid mucous,** having the smell of rotten cheese. Hypersensitiveness to cold, to touch, to contrariety (irascible character). Coryza, rhino-pharyngitis, false croup, trachea-bronchitis, hypertrophy of tonsils. Used generally in all catarrhal inflammation of respiratory system, specially of the larynx and trachea in scrofulous subjects. Children with short neck having tendency to spasms of glotis, easily suffocated (F. Bernoville).

Idoium—Clear discharge with swelling of the mucous membranes. Excoriation Crusts and obstruction of the nose, loss of smell, aggravation by cold, dry and painful cough (the childs holds its laryns) preferably in the morning. Hepatisation of the right lung, upper lobe. Fever with chill, great internal and external heat. Redness of the cheeks, agitation. Great thirst with abundant sweat, Adenitis, croyza, trachea-bronchitis, pneumonia, pleuritis, tracheobronchial adenopathy.

Ipecac—Naso-pharyngial catarrh in fat and chubby child. It may be used in two ways in cough. Lower dilutions 3x & 6 act like an expectorant, fluidifies the bronchial mucous and of the alveolus and favours elimination. In high dilution, 30, it acts as antispasmodic and stops expectoration. A very important remedy which is to be applied in violent suffocating cough. The bronchi are full of mucous, the face is bluish. There is persistent nausea with vomiting which soes not ameliorate nausea; often diarrhoea with watery and greenish stools.

The tongue is clear. Laryngo-trachitis. **Bronchitis, whooping cough, pneumonia,** capillary bronchitis, asthma, hemoptysis.

Kali bichormicum—Viscous, thready nasal catarrh having the tendency to become localised in the rhino-pharynx. Pain in the root of the nose at the place of sinus. Hard, greenish, ball like mucous difficult to detach. Often there is ulceration after expulsion. Scraping cough, yellowish expectoration, abundant in the form of stingy filamen, difficult to expectorate and which can be seen extending from the throat. Amelioration in the heat of the bed. Sinusitis, **rhino-phary-ngitis,** bronchitis, whooping cough. It is besides a remedy with **Pulsatilla,** to be applied when the acute diseases of the respiratory system are on the decrease (bronchitis, whooping cough, pneumonia) when the cough and expectoration do not ameliorate at par with the general symptoms.

Kali carbonicum—Lymphatic children, **less resistant, chilly, easily fatigued.** Cough with transfixing thoracic pain, localised at the base of the right lung. Aggravation by movement. Chronic cough with bad general condition as a consequence of an acute affection of the respiratory system. **Aggravation by cold. Amelioration of all symptoms while bending forward.**

Kali iodatum—Abundant discharge from the eyes and nose. Irritating discharge with sneezing. Raucous cough with dyspnoea, oedema of the larynx. Amelioration of general symptoms **in open air,** but aggravation of the Coryza. Syphilitic ground. Acute Coryza, teachitis, bronchitis.

Lycopodium—Crust and obstruction of the nostrils causing the patient to sleep with open mouth. Chronic thick discharge. Dry cough with dyspnoea, aggravation from 4 to 8 p. m. Fanning of the nostrils. Fever with chill followed by sweat. Small pulse, general condition is bad, great irritability. The child becomes angry if one approaches it, thwarts its encourage and cries. Cough with greet expectoration, with the tendency of becoming chronic after pneumonia. Long lasting, dragging broncho-pneumonia changing seats.

Mercurius solubilis—Watery, irritating nasal flow with photophobia, worse in hot room. Stinging pain of the tonsils, of the pharynx which are red. Tendency to excoriation and ulceration of the nostrils. Cough worse at night with abundant sweats having bad smell, **which does not ameliorate. Humid tongue,** salvation, great thirst for cold water. A good remedy of Coryza often the stage of *Belladonna*.

Mercurius Corrosives—Same modalities as that of *Merc sol*, but irritation, photophobia, excoriation are more marked.

Phosphorus—Horseness worse in the morning. Cough with burning in the larynx, sensation of heaviness behind the sternum. Aggravation by cold. Painful points in the chest. Fever with chill without thirst with red and dry tongue. **Pharynx red and dry,** varnished, loaded with adhesive mucous.

Sensation of burning, spasms and suffocation. Rusty expectoration. Rapid pulse with accelerated respiration, fanning of nostrils. It is the most important remedy of pneumonia and broncho-pneuhapatisation begins. Its action is centrifugal and it often causes the absorption of the exudation in 38 or 48 hours. If its action is complete we should wait for two days and then we should repeat it. One of the best remedies of **Infantile Asthma.**

Pneumonia broncho-pneumonia, pulmonary congestion, **asthma**. It is dangerous in tuberculosis.

Pulsatilla—It is indicated **in the period of efferves-cence** of an acute affection of the respiratory system when **there is easy cough with abundant and sweetish expec-toration. Aggravation in a hot room**. (Viscous, thready expectoration better in hot room (*Kali bich.*) In some chronic catarrhs with thick yellowish sputum; **loss of smell,** with nasal obstruction, amelioration in open air. Finally because of its deep anti-tubercular action, it is often used during convalescence after acute infections in children.

Rhus toxicodendron—Rhino-pharynigitis influenza after being exposed to **humid cold. Adynamic form of influenza** or of some broncho-pneumonia with dry tongue, covered with a dark coating, with triangle at the tip of the tongue. Great thirst, agitation at night. Stupor, mild deliriums, mutterings. Dry skin, hot, often with abundant sweats. Dark-red face.

Rumex crispus—An interesting remedy of trachitis. In-cessant violent cough, **aggravation by cold wind by pres-sure in the sternal hollow** pickling of trachea causing cough. Amelioration by heat, in a hot room. Persons who cough by the least cold will always try to keep himself hotly dressed, even the head well covered.

Sabadilla—Nasal discharge with noisy sneezing, fre-quent, spasmodic. The pricking in the nose often passes from the right to the left. **Amelioration by head,** drinking hot water of drinks. Aggravation in open air, during full moon. It is remedy of Coryza of spasmodic type It may check an asthmatic attack that begins from the nose. Coryza **has fever, asthma.**

Sambucus—An important remedy of spasmodic affections of the respiratory system. Suffocating cough, coming suddenly towards midnight; dryness and obstruction of the nose and sudden suffocation. The child wakes up in a start, sits up on the bed, **has the need for fresh air.** Cannot breathe, face becomes violet. Fever with profuse sweat. It is afraid of being uncovered. Bad temperament, anxiety. Better while sitting on the bed by movement. **False croup asthma.**

Sangunaria condenses—Great sensitiveness to smell (of flowers) Abundant, corrosive Coryza, that becomes thick and may stop, giving rise to diarrhoea. Right sidedness. with burning pain in the conjunctiva. Continual weakning cough with **burning sensation** in the chest, oppression, constriction. Aggravation at night. Circumscribed redness of the face, often one sided (**Cham**), distension of temporal veins. Rusty sputa. Feets are burning, searches for cold place, Amelioration in **fresh air**. Pulmonary congestion, pneumonia (right sided), **asthma.**

Silicea—Catarrhal affections of the respiratory system of children who are tubercular of sycotic. Chronic sequences of **acute suppurative diseases,** abcess of the lungs, purulent pleuresy. Should be given at the end of these **affections to stop the suppuration** or the check a fistula.

Tuberculosis with purulent expectoration. Hectic fever, with sweats. Asthma. Aggravation by cold. Better by covering (even the head).

Spongia tosta—Larynx dry, sensitive with a sensation of constriction and burning. Continual cough aggravation in the evening. Tickling in the trachea. Suffocating cough aggravation at night by heat, by **bending the head.** Better sitting, drinking hot water. It is a very important remedy of false croup. It is very important remedy of cough, false croup, trachitic asthma. **Recurrent cough.**

Stannum—Hoarseness. Fits of cough of **weak subjects,** aggravation while speaking, laughing and **drinking**. Purulent expectoration like white of eggs having sweet taste. Sensation of emptiness in the chest. Profuse night sweats. Cachexia, **tuberculosis.**

Sticta pulmonialis—Sneezing. Painful sensation of pressure and **fullness at the root of the nose**. Rhino-pharyngitis, asthma.

Sulphur—**It is an important remedy of centrifugal action**. It is indicated at the beginning of the acute diseases of children. Should be used in 30th potency. It very often checks the course of the disease and cures the disease. It is preferable not to give it during the evolution of the affection.

After the defervescence when convalescence has begun, it is to be used to eliminate the toxins and to check the tendency to Chronicity and to avoid morbid metastasis and complication. *Sulphur* 30 or 200 should be given anew in all acute infections of infancy. When there is the fear of aggravation in less resistant tubercular child it is to be substituted by *Sulphur iodaatum.*

Inspite of the value of Homoeopathic medicines and the excellent results obtained it is often necessary to add with them some Nosodes in the affection of the respiratory system of infants.

The selection of Nosodes are based less on their pathogenesis then on their general clinical symptoms and the ideas that we have about the epidemic in question. At the beginning of influenza it is necessary to prescribe *Influenzum* 30. But we must know that it will act according to the seasonal character of the epidemic. It is for this reason we get prepared different stocks at the beginning of the epidemic and experience has taught us that a stock which was curative in the month of November was not efficacious in March.

Pyrogenium—Excellent remedy in grave cases of influenza or in **pneumopathy.** Septicemia is feared. *Pyrogenium* is a nosode prepared from putrid meat in trituration, administered in 30 or 200. It is a remedy of great value. It is generally clinically applied to grave states of the type of

Arsenicum which it follows very successfully. **Dissociation of pulse and temperature.** But it may be applied even without this symptom. it is remedy which has helped in cases of mastoiditis and it has cured many cased of influenza, pneumonia, bronchopneumonia of grave types. We should make delay for its application.

Marmoreck, Aviary, Bacillinum are used when the remedies indicated do not give satisfactory results in pneumonia and in bronchopneumonia.

Pertussin—At the beginning use 30th and during convalescence use 100 or 200. A useful method communicated to us by Roche (de Poille) consists in applying *Pertussin* 30 & *Sulphur* 30 alternately ever five days. We have tried it and have found very useful.

Nux vomica—Coryza **after cold and humid weather** with nasal obstruction, heaviness at the root of the nose. Watery discharge during the day which **stops at night** in a hot room with sensation of dryness in the nose. Hypersensitiveness to smell. Cough aggravates towards 3 to 5 A. M. by **inhalation of cold air,** by exercise, while eating. Amelioration by heat, rest and by hot drinks.

Coryza, sinusitis, rhino-pharyngits.

To illustrate the theoretical ideas, we have selected from our case book of acute infantile pulmonary affection some cases. Here is a summary.

CASE REPORTS

I

Girl P., 3 years.

On my return from a journey, the doctor who was working in my place informed me that he is very much anxious about a girl since four days. The girl is suffering from a grave form of bronchopneumonia. I knew the child, who last winter was attacked by the same disease and I had great difficulty to cure her.

I found the following symptoms: high fever, small, rapid theready pulse. Paleness of the face and cyanosis of the extremities, general coldness, cold sweats. Fanning of the nostrils. Nausea, incontinence of stools and urine. By auscultation, the two lungs are full of rales of all types, the seats of the rales have the character of gurgling. The cough has become rare, expectoration impossible. Thirst for cold water. Complete anorexia. The parents have lost one girl who suffered from bronchopneumonia three years ago.

On the mothers side there is the history of serious tubercular antecedents: a brother had been discharged from military service and was given pension because of a double pleuropneumonial congestion, followed by sero-fibrinous pleurecy of the right lung. Had since then condensation of the lung and asthma in the winter. Two brothers died of tubercular meningitis when young. The mother herself suffered from repeated bronchitis, had slight attack of asthma at the age between 16 to 20 years. Had suppurated adenitis in the second infancy. If I believe in the antecedents, I thought the prognosis should be grave.

Prescriptions: *Animonium tartaricum* 30, two granules very three hours.

On the following day, slight amelioration of the appearance and of the general symptoms. Stethoscopic symptoms are stationary.

Aviary 100 one dose.

Antimonium tartaricum, 30 every three hours.

Immediate amelioration. I replace Antimonium tartaricum *by Ipecac* 6, alternated every two hours with *Bryonia.*

The fever subsided. The condition of the heart is better. Auscultation reveals a considerable diminution of the rales, the child expectorated while vomiting; grayish sputum, having a bad smell. It can sit up on the bed alone and asks for food. It is irritable, pushes its mother and the doctor. *Lycopodium* 30 is added to *Ipecac* and *Bryonia,* one dose in the evening.

Two days after, the girl is in full convalescence. *Pulsatilla* 6, *Sulphur iodatum* 6, are prescribed for five days. Cure without further complication.

Inspite of the gravity of the case I made a strict

homoeopathic treatment without the help of a cardiac tonic, of a colloidal metal or injections of oxygen.

II

A child of 13 months, male, of a camp. March 1931.

The child is suffering from asphyxia; it was in a deplorable hygienic condition: in a poor filthy condition, in an icy barrack open on all sides. The mother refuses to hospitalise it. Generalised capillary bronchitis. Cold sweats, collapse, liquid diarrhoea with incontinence. Death seemed inevitable.

Carbo vegetabillis 30, to be taken as early as possible.

Camphora 6, to be taken every hour.

Antimonium crudum 30 every two hours.

Next morning the child has better respiration. Same treatment.

In the evening the fever rises, but the respiratory condition is clearly better. Some coughs with small expectoration. Agitation alternating with prostration. Thirst for small quantity of cold water.

Aviary 100 one dose.
Ipecac 6.
Arsenicum album 30.
Bryonia 6.

Progressive amelioration. Cure within four days.

III

A child of 6 months, male. February, 1932.

Parentsame to my chamber after 19Km of journey, in an insufficiently closed coach. The child was covered in heaps of covers, Snow was falling since two days, penetrating cold, eastern wind.

They informed that since the morning the child has $40^0.5$ fever, that it is coughing and suffocating. The child is agitated, burning with fixed eyes. I scolded the parents for having subjected the child to make such a long journey in snowy weather. Their answer was that they wanted their child to be treated by me and they found no other way but to come directly to me.

By auscultation: Tubular sound of the base of the right lung with some crepitant rales. I told my diagnosis to the parents and I prescribed.

Aconite 6, two granules every two hours.

I saw the child next day at noon. Temperature $38^0.2$. The rale is more soft, tubular sound is diminished. Cough nausea.

Ipecac
Phosphorus 30

The next day the temperature is $3^0.5$. Cure in 43 hours.

IV

Girl, 11 months. December 1932.

Broncho-pneumonia both sides affected. Familial tuberculinism. Pauperism. Bad hygienic condition: psycological misery. Slight fever (loss of defense reaction), small pulse, rapid. Prostration and delirium. Weak cough, superficial respiration. Fanning of the nostrils.

External coldness. I had not great hope to cure the child.

Treatment: *Pyrogenium* 30
Phosphorus 30
Antimonium tartaricum 3x.

The next day, the condition is stationary: however the pulse has become more rapid. The child is less prostrated.

Treatment: *Antimonium tartaricum* 3x.
Arsenic 30

Progressive amelioration. Two days after I repeated *Phosphorus* 30 and replaced *Antimonium* by *Ipecac* and now *Arsenic* 30 once a day and in a week I obtained the cure.

Treatment during the convalescence: *Arsenicum iodatum*, *Pulsatilla* and later on *Marmoreck*.

V

Child of 2 and a half month, male. November 1932. Breast fed.

Familial tubercular and syphilitic antecedents. Fifteen days ago series of asthmatic fits. Child is punny, pale, nervous and does not sleep. Chill while changing clothes after a diarrhoea. Capillary bronchitis with suffocation, violet colour of the face, agitation, want of air.

Treatment: *Sambucus* 3x, gtt. III every two hours.
Antimonium tartaricum 30, 2 granules every two hours.
Marmoreck 30 one dose.

The child struggles between life and death for 48 hours, then his condition becomes better. The symptoms of capillary bronchitis diminished, but at night towards 1 O'clock it has fits of asthma with suffocation.

Treatment: *Sambucus* 1x.
Arsenicum album 30
Ipecac 6.

The fits diminished and finally disappeared after a week. I continued the treatment for 3 months and I was able to avoid all dangerous pathological conditions.

VI

A girl 7 months. December, 1932.

A young mother came to me and told me with tears the following facts: her baby of 7 months (mixed feeding) was attacked with whooping cough clearly confirmed since about 10 days. Treatment: Vaccines (neo-dmetys, Clin's Vaccine) and soothing potious. Since four days, a broncho-pneumonia is declared. Three doctors met and they declared that the child was lost, and gave no prescription. At one glance I found that the condition of the child is what one calls "It has only last breath of life". Coma, closed eyelids, pale with spots of cyanosis, preagonical coldness. It seemed that the child will lose its last breath by the slightest movement. Told the mother to take the child in arms so that I may examine it. Temperature 30^0. Imperceptible pulse cannot be counted. Short, jerky respiration. Bilateral bronchopneumonia with multiple points of hepatisation of different maturity. Excessively rapid heart. Embryo Cardiac rythme. I confirmed the prognosis of my colleagues and said to the mother that the child is moribund. Perhaps I will not be of any help. Nevertheless I did my duty and prescribed the homoeopathic remedy of agony *Carbo vegetabilis* 200 dose. I told the mother to inform me next morning if the child was not dead. Early in the next morning I was called in the phone and was told: Doctor please come soon, my baby is living, it is moving its feet. The child seemed in fact less moribund. It is covered with cold sweats, it was moving its lips. Respiration seemed deeper when the mother fans it. It has sipped a few drops of water.

I repeat *Carbo vegetabilis* 30, accompanied by *Camphora* 6 one dose.

In the evening the child opened its eyes: it is very much violet, slight cough. Temperature 38.5.

Treatment: *Antimonium tartaricum* 200 one dose.

Carbo vegetablis is stopped.

On the following day apparent amelioration. The child opens its eyes, moves, its extremities, drinks some water and mother's milk. Loss cyanosed, less asphyxiated.

Prescription: *Antimonium tartaricum* 30 every two hours.

In the evening, temperature is 39^0. I told the mother that the child is saved because I found that with better febril reaction, there is amelioration of all the symptoms. Added to my treatment:

Arsenic 30, one dose.
Pertussin 30, one dose the following day.

The whooping-cough appeared. Auscultation revealed some signs of bronchitis. The fits of whooping-cough are 20 during 24 hours. The child vomited mucous.

Treatment: *Ipecac* 3x.
   Corallia 6.

The fever falls. Everything goes well. There is no more any question of bronchopneumonia and in eight days the whooping cough is cured.

VII

Child, 3 years. Male. December 1932.

The neighbour of the above child came to see me for the same pathological conditions. A whooping-cough mal-treated by vaccination for three weeks. No more prescription, for hygienic adjuvant, becomes complicated with broncho-pneumonia. The condition is less grave than that of the preceding case. It is a child of two years, robust with a massive seat blocking the whole lower lobe of the right lung. It has suffocation and is completely asphyxiated. Lying on its back, cyanosed, with dilated pupils, froth in the mouth, complete incontinence of stools and urine. Temperature 41°. It was an evening towards 6 O'clock. I prescribed *Antimonium tartaricum* 200, one dose. The following day at 11, I saw the patient. It was lying calm and breathing more freely. After the dose of Antimonium tart it vomited a great quantity of mucous, thick, mixed with frothy matter. Temperature 39°. Treatment *Ipecac* 6.

The following day at the same hour, the child was sitting up on the bed and asks for eating, drinking and trying to stand up. Temperature 37°.5. General condition perfect.

Auscultation reveals numerous humid rales at the base of the lung. Almost complete absorption of the seat. The whooping cough which became weakly reactive was cured in a week.

After one month I was called urgently for the same

patient. It has cold, having escaped from the maternal care and without being properly dressed, in the dry cold weather. Temperature $40^0.5$. Redness of the face, thirst, agitation, Auscultation: tubular sound at the base of the right lung. No rales.

Treatment: *Aconite* 6, every two hours.

The next day the temperature is $37^0.5$. The sound disappeared within 48 hours. No more complication.

Conclusion

We have said that we have selected from among our cases, those that are more interesting and grave. Personally I have the custom to relate not only my successes but also my failures. As regards the field of the disease of the respiratory system of infants, we should say, that during our three last years of practice we had not the occasion to deplore a single death. We have no kept a mathematical statistics of our cases but we think that among more than one hundred cases there was not even a single failure. At the beginning of our homoeopathic practice we never regretted for being faithful to homoeopathy. We were particularly impressed by the quality of results which encouraged us to learn carefully and completely the Materia Medica, in order to become better therapeutists.

Finally le me summarise the advantages of homoeopathy in the treatment of pulmonary diseases of infants.

1. Foresee and prevent the disease, knowing the ground.

2. Treatment with the maximum chance of success.

3. Treating the convalescence, avoid the metastasis, and morbid transfer and prepare for a future of excellent health.

4. Homoeopathy helps to possess a general theoretical idea and practical as well, in order to formulate a prognosis with maximum accuracy.

REMEDIES OF THE RESPIRATORY SYSTEM

A topographical representation

1. Upper Respiratory tract

(a) Lacrymal gland and Lacrymal duct

Guarea—A capital remedy of dacryocystitis with obstruction of the lacrymal duct. Less known remedy, but very much used by DR. Parteneau in 1x. It acts specially in **dacryocystitis, acute or chronic.** Dr. Bernoville prescribes in granules, two granules once a day. Corresponding ground remedies are very often: *Thuja Lachesis, Lycopodium, Hepar Sulphur (Suppurated dacryocystitis).*

(b) Nasal mucous and cavum

1. *Acute Coryza. Allium cepa, Euphrasia, Arsenic, Mercurius,*

Pulsatilla—with sometimes *Hepar sulphur* form the small group of remedies of acute rhinitis.

Allium cepa—Irritating nasal flow, irritating lacrymation. These two remedies may be alternated. They are also indicated in the catarrhal phase in the beginning of measles and in hay asthma were it should be used in the 30th, repeated every day, often simultaneously with 1000 in long intervals (Nebel).

Arsenicum album is opposite of *Mercurius. Arsenic:* acute coryza with catarrh directed towards the exterior with red nostrils; great irritation of the mucous membranes and even of the upper lip. Amelioration by hot applications. *Mercurius:* catarrh directed to wards the interior, towards the pharynx, with possible erythematous angina. First stage of suppuration, the second stage is marked by *Hepar sulphur* and the third stage (chronic stage) by *Silicea.*

Pulsatilla—Used at the end of the acute stage when the flow is yellow, non-irritating and sweet.

All these remedies play an important role only in the acute stage of coryza but also in the treatment of sinusitis.

II. Chronic Rhinitis

Hydrastis and Kali bichromicum have almost similar indications: **Thick yellow thready discharge.** They may be used together because they reinforce the actions of each other. When the nasal discharge requires increasing, they are to be used in lower dilutions 3 and 6, for Hydrastis, 6 and 12 *Kali bich.* On the contrary when the stoppage of the discharge is necessary the 30th dilution is to be used. Let us insist on the symptom of *Kali bichr.:* thick, elastic, greenish yellow crusts, thrown out of the nose when the patient sneezes.

Kali muriaticum and Kali iodatum—They act in chronic nontherady nasal discharge. Lump of mucous difficult to detach in *Kali mur.* with whitish discharge. Action on the eustachianube. In **Kali** iod. the discharge is very fluid, like the white of an egg. colorless and very much abundant.

We know that the upper respiratory tract, particularly the cavum, formes a real cross-road between the different bony stages of the face and between the digestive and the respiratory apparatus which explains the, existence, from physiopatholgical point of view, the naso **hepatic syndromes, naso intestinal symptoms** like that of **naso urinary syndromes or naso genital syndromes. It is a capital rule in Homoeopathic Drainage to search what is the other pole of the organism: Which has the nasal pole for the toxinic equilibrium.** The nose is undoubtedly an emonoctory of derivation, which is the most used by the human organism. Unfortunately we have not yet any sure rule by which we can envisage in a clear manner the syndrome in question. Perhaps one may think of the right passage of the cavum when the liver is the cause. The right nostril is particularly affected. We may think of the urinary and the genital apparatuses when the cavum and nose are affected bilaterally. But this fact remains to be elucidated.

The most important fact to note: when *Lycopodium* is the ground remedy (hepatic insufficiency), the elimination is marked through the right nostril. The second interesting point: In the pathogenesis of the remedies having elective actions on the liver, we note always the symptoms of pharyngitis (*Chelidonium, Chionanthus, China and Myrica*). The third example is of the same nature: Some remedies like *Agrentum nitricum and* **Capsicum** always respond to a balance between the urinary and genital apparatus and the nasal mucous membranes, such as it is seen in some cases of acute *rhinokpharyngitis* with *albuminuria*. We have already had the occasion to stress on the point that, the idea of elective action of medicines and their polarity of action dominate the importance of drainage and of canalisation. Dr. Rouy has begun a research in this sense. He has been able to show that in some cases, such part of the *crystalline* was related to such remedy which should orient the mind towards such to be of the liver.

III. Pharyngitis

If we have to draw a chart of the remedies of diphtheria we will indicate;

Lachesis—Elective action on the left tonsil. *Lachesis* is very important.

With *Arsentic*, it is the remedy of serious infections in general, even gangrenous.

Mercurius cyanatus—It is the most effective salts of mercury.

Mercurius proto-odatus—It has an affinity for the right tonsil and *Mercurius biodatus* for the left.

We have still other important remedies such as *Apis* (Oedema of the uvula) and *Kali bichromicum*, which we have already studied.

Some other remedies have action specially on the glottis. *Hepar sulphur* is classic. Dr. Bernoville says that it acts better in children having short neck, the head being pressed between the shoulders. **They have tendency to spasm of glottis.** *Apis* is an important remedy of the oedema of the uvula. Then come *Cantharis* and *Arsenic* and in the case where the oedema of glottis is caused by be sting, we must think of *Ledum palustre* and *Calendula*.

IV. Laryngitis

The most important and dominating remedy is *Drosera,* which is used in all sorts of laryngial phenomena in relation to a tubercular state. it should be given in rather high dilution 200, but rarely repeated and with great care because its action is like that of *Phosphorus* and that of *Tuberculines.* On our schema we have drawn an arrow downwards vertically and we have indicated *Sambucus* the mucous falls in the throat which causes the spasm of the glottis). We have drawn an ascending arrow and we have indicated Bromium *(of which the mucous* has a tandency towards the exterior), a remedy of laryngo-trachitis and of *Asthma* ameliorating on the sea side. It is also a remedy extending to larynx and to the trachea. On the point of the sternal fork, the most important remedy is *Rumex crispus,* acting specially on the lower part of the larynx and trachea. The **cough**

is caused by pressure above the fork, or while breathing cold air. it is better used in **tubercular condition** and to patients of oxygenoid constitution, who may have diarrhea towards the morning like that of the *Sulphur* type.

Hyoscyamus has cough with congestion of the brain in horizontal position with the impression that the uvula is tickling on the posterior part of the pharynx. These troubles disappear in a vertical position. *Hyoscyamus* is a remedy of **pharyngeal cough** like that of *Capsicum* (sensation of burning with the menace of otitis) and *Mentha piperita* (the patient has the sensation of swallowing cold air, and cold air aggravates). It is equally a remedy of trachitis (aggravation at night in lying position) like that of *Rumex crispus*. Finally *Hyoscymus*, *Kali bich* and *Apis* from the trio having elective action on the uvula.

With *Bromium* and *Rumex* we may compare *Chlorum*, *Ammonium iodatum*, *Ammonicacum*, which are the remedies of the secondary importance.

Sulphur is our important polychrest. It should not be neglected in laryngo-trached cough.

In recurrent cough, nervous cough of cardiac origin let us think of *Naja* and *Spongia*. We must not forget *igitalis* (action on the heart).

Let us now consider a series of remedies having special action on the larynx.

Aconite, Spongia and *Hepar* sulphur, the classic trio of

croupal cough. *Aconite* and *Spongia* have croupal cough at nigh. *Hepar after* midnight. *Aconite* has much anxiety *Spongia* has noisy cough, having sawing sound. We may use *Aconite* and *Spongia* 6 alternately every four hours and *Hepar sulphur* once in 24 hours. Use the 30th potency.

Arum triphyllum is specially indicated in the acute stage and even in grave stages of secondary streptococcus infection. The patient has very much nasal voice, bi-tonal voice, and continually pricks his lips and tears the skin.

The remedies of chronic laryngitis are related to *Carbo vegetabilis*, *Phosphorus* and *Causticum* as ground remedies.

Phosphorus—It is the remedy of congestive or inflammatory stages. Hoarseness in the evening, after overwork of the voice which causes congestion of the larynx. *Phosphorus* is the *Bryonia* of larynx.

Causticum is the remedy of paresis and of atony. Its hoarseness is worse in the morning; *Causticum* acts on the motility of the larynx. *Causticum* is the *Rhus tox* of the larynx.

We know that *Causticum* and *Phosphorus* are incompatible.

Carbo vegetabilis is an important remedy having elective action on the larynx. We should think of it in all cases of acute laryngitis or of chronic laryngitis specially when all other remedies have failed, or have caused the acute stage to enter into chronic stage. There is at the same time atony and congestion. But the congestion is more passive than inflammatory. The patient has a sensation of heat or even burning in the larynx and trachea. Aphonia is often complete. There is the possibility of cyanosis and hyposphyxia.

Carbo veg. is related to *Arnica* and *Selenium* which are its complementary.

In the laryngitis of influenza. laryngeal cough, catarrhal laryngitis with incessant cough, it is always better not to wait for the search of simillimum. It is better to use the more sure remedies alternately. As for example we may prescribe *Drosera* 200, one dose, followed every hour by *Sambucus* 6, *Runex 6,* and *Spongia* 6. We will thus have a good and rapid result.

Cuprum metallicum is an important antispasmodic remedy, specially useful in whooping cough or in whooping-cough-like cough with possible cyanosis and laryngeal suffocation (like *Carbo vegetabilis*). Amelioration by drinking cold water (like *Causticum*).

Coralium rubrum is the opposite of *Cuprum.* The child becomes red during the fit of whooping-cough. Really speaking *Cuprum* acts also very well, even if the child becomes red during the fit.

Let us recall here some of the principal remedies of

whooping cough: *Belladonna, Ipecac, Drosera, Coccus cacti, Mephitis, Arnica, Cina* and the Nosode *Pertussin.*

These are the principal remedies having an elective action on the larynx and trachea. Let us now consider the remedies having a local elective action on the bronchi, the lungs and the pleura.

II. Lower Respiratory system

1. Pleuresy and pleuritis.

Seven remedies are of the first importance: *Sulphur iodatum,* which is the most important of all. Its satellite is *Arsencium iodatum;* then the trio of pleuresy: *Bryonia, Ramunculus bulbosus, Asclepias tuberosa;* finally the duo of the exudation: *Cantharis* and *Apis,* do which we may add *Kali carbonicum.*

Sulphur iodum is indicated in pleuritis for avoiding pleuresy. In course of pleuresy, to check symphysis, and finally when there is symphysis. It is also indicated in *Cortico-pleuritis. Sulphur idoum,* acts rather on the left lung, while *Phosphorus triodatus* acts rather on the right.

Arsenicum iodum has the same indications as that of *Sulphur iod.* It is an excellent remedy in general, in oxygeniod tubercularis patient, more or less menaced by pulmonary bacillosis. Has special action on the right lung.

Bryonia is the most important of the three remedies of pleuritis. Pains ameliorated by rest, aggravated by movement. Right sided.

Ranunculus bulbosus: Pleurodonia aggravated by humidity. Left laterality. Marked action in rheumatic and alcoholic patients in relation to *Lalchesis and Sulphur.*

Asclepia tuberosa ; Tubercular condition. Acts specially on the left base.

Cantharis and *Apis* are the remedies of exudation. *Cantharis* being the most important.

Kali carb is a remineralising remedy. Should be applied at the end of pleuresy.

One point merits special mention here. Opposition between *Sulphur iodatun* and *Phosphorus. Phosphorus triodatus* is more indicated in tubercular patients having central pulmonary lesions of caseous type, while *Sulphur iodatum* responds to peripheric fibro-caseous or fibrous lessions.

Finally let us not forget the remarkable decongestive action of *Sepia* on the left apex. *Sepia* is an important remedy but the most misunderstood remedy of tuberculosis and of congestion of the left apex. When one treats a recalcitrant tuberculous patient, when it does not react to medicines and seems to evolve towards an evaluative phase, with a left apical localisation, we must think of *Sepia,* even in the absence of the general symptoms of the remedy.

II. Pulmonary and bronchial affections.

Lycopodium and *Chelidonium* act on the right base purely topographically, affecting the whole inferior portion of the hemithorax (right) (right lobe of the liver, pleural cul-de-sac, base of the right lung). It is opposed to *Sulphur, Natrum sulphuricum, Antimonium sulphuricum auratum* acting specially on left base in asthma.

Bryonia is indicated from the pulmonary point of view. It acts specially on the right lung.

Antimoninm tartaricum acts on the two lungs, like *Ipecac, Antimonium* is one of the most faithful remedy of expectoration. Elective action on the bronchial mucous and on the bronchial alveoles. Has also action on the heart. On the contrary *ipecac* acts through the medium of the vagus on the diaphragm and on the bronchial mucous. It acts very well on the respiratory spasms and bronchial mucous. But it may cause congestion if it is given very often or in very high dilutions.

Ethyl sulphuricum discoloratum is the remedy of the acute oedema of the lungs. Satellite of *Phosphours* and of *Sulphur.*

Phosphorus is here an important remedy of pulmonary congestions, of bronchopneumonia and of pneumonia, action selectively on the parenchyma, of the lungs, specially on the right side.

Silicea is opposed to Phosphorus. It acts on the intersti-
tial pulmonary tissues, on the pulmonary elasticity. It is a
remedy of suppuration, and a remedy of emphysema as well
(metabolical trouble of silicate on the lengs). In persons
suffering from emphysema one will often give *Phosphorus*
and *Silicea* alternately in high dilutions. *Phosphorus* during
congestive phases. *Silicea* for giving more elasticity.

We will not speak here again about different antispasmodic remedies such as *Cuprum, Ipecac, Hydrocyanic acid*
etc., which we have already studied. We will speak only
about those that have elective action. *Phellandrium:* pain
which crosses the right apex; *Myrtus communis* on the right
apex: *Illicium,* pain specially on the third rib of the right side
and of the corresponding cartilage; *Chelidonium:* spontane-
ous pain, one or two centimeters below the lower angle of
the right shoulder blade. *Chenopod glauciaphs* has similar
pain on the left shoulder blade.

And let us now conclude our study by some general
consideration about the important ground remedies (Schema
II): *Sulphur, Phosphorus, Arsenic* and *Carbo vegetabilis.*

Sulphur is used specially in congestive stages, but the
remedy has a centrifugal action. It is used at the end of the
acute stage.

Phosphorus is also a remedy of congestive states, but as

the action of the remedy is centripetal it should be manipulated rightly.

Arsenic is indicated when the patient has lost his vitality.

Carbo *vegetabilis* is used when there is a greater loss of the vital force.

Often the respiratory troubles evolves according to these four remedies, i.e. to say one may check the gravest (*Carbo veg*) and less grave (*Sulphur*).

On the each side of our schema we may indicate: *Lachesis*, the great remedy of hyposphyxic conditions, *Igantia*, *Cimicifuga*, *Cuprum* are the remedies of spasms. On the left of our table and on the top:

Lycopodium, pneumonia of children with fanning of the nostrils: *Nux vomica* its complementary: *Thuja* and *Natrum sulphuricum*, remedies of hydrogeniod constitution and of sycosis, opposed to psoric conditions of all the other remedies of the chart; *Sepia*, a remedy of the respiratory system, though it is less important, yet it should not be neglected; it is related to *Nux vomica* and *Thyja*. *Causticum*, a remedy of aphonia, laryngial paresis, is related to *Thuja* and *Natrum Sulphuricum*.

Psorinum is very important in pulmonary affections specially chronic and responds to chronic *Sulphur* aggravated while evolving towards *Carbo veg*. and *Opium* (uremia).

Silicea and *Phosphorus* are opposed to each other, *Silicea* is related to *Natrum muriaticum* which follows *Natrum Sulphuricum.* Between *Sulphur* and *Iodium* is placed *Sulphur iodatum,* which is very important in tuberculinics. The adolescent *Natrum muriaticum* which evolves towards *Silicea,* may have pulmonary lesions of serious functional troubles which may evolve towards *Sepia* or *Lachesis.* The patients of *Sepia* and *Lachesis* are often chronic *Natrum muriaticum* or chronic *Pulsatilla. Natrum muriaticum* has also important relations with *Calcarea carbonica* and with its complementary *Hepar sulphur,* a remedy of supurations (pulmonary), which may later on evolve towards *Silicea.* We may still indicate some satellites of these polychrests *Ipium* and *Morphinum,* remedies of uremic coma. *Around Opium: Cuprum arsenicosum* (spasms), *Ammonium carbonicum Carbolic acid, Helleborus.*

Carbolic acid, Helleborus, Opium and *Morphimum* are the four remedies of Cheyne-Stockes respiration.

Between *Phosphorus* and *Carbo veg.: Cuprum* and *Veratrum album.* Let us also think of the trio of vegotonia: *Ipecac, Hydrocyanic acid, Lobelia inflate.*

Silicea has some relations with *Baryta carbonicum* in pulmonary sclerosis.

Pulsatilla is an important drainer of *Phosphorus, Sulphur* and *Lycopodium.*

Rhus toxicodendron, the drainer of *Thuja* and *Natrum Sulphuricum*.

We find also the three important remedies of the drainage of Dr. ebel's tuberculinic: *Pulsatilla, drainer of*Marmoreck; *Rhustox*, drainer of *T. R. and Denys; Nux vomica*, dainer of T. K. Some times T. R. and the hydrogenoid conditions are drained by *Nux vomica* and *Ipecac*.

Sulphur's important satellite in acute cases: *Aconite*.

PSORA

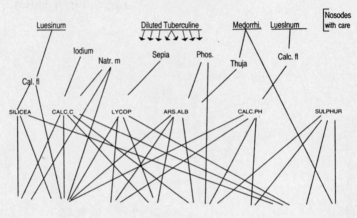

Luesinum   Iodium   Natr. m   Diluted Tuberculine   Sepia   Phos.   Medorrhi.   Luesinum   Nosodes with care

Cal. fl   Thuja   Calc. fl

SILICEA   CALC.C   LYCOP   ARS.ALB   CALC.PH   SULPHUR

Athrepsia	Tr of	Anoerxia	Vomitting	Diarrhoea	Colics	Constipation		Skin tr
Congenital	growth	(Mental)	Dyspepsia	Cholera				
Weakness	Rickets	Liver tr	Indigestion	Infantile				
Anemia	Leanness	Acetonemia		Etericolitis				
	Obesity							
Abroat.	Baryta	Ipecac	Ipecac	Greendiarr	Cholera	Chamm.	Bryonia	Chamm.
Ars. iod.	Sul. iod	Antim.c	Aethusa	Arg. nit.	Veratr.	Bellad.	Farax.	Bellad.
Calc. sil	Oleum	Lecithine	Antim.c	Ipecac	Antim.c	China	Calc. acet.	Rhus. tox
Acetic. ac	Ars. iod	Puls		Aconlte	Cuprum m	Coloc.	Graph.	Arnica
Ferr. met	Kali. iod	Senna	I	Bellad.	Campi.	Ver. alb	Opium	Cantharis
Puls.	Dur. met		Iris vers			Diosco	Alumin	
	Vitamins		Mercdul		Clear diarr		Mag. m	Local care
	Organotheraphy		Senna	Mag. c	Chain			Calenduls
				Rheum.	Podo.			
				Kreosot.	China			
				Aethusa				

Other remedies
Merc. sol.   Painless
Merc. cor   [Diarrhoea
Merc. dul   Phos. ac
Bryon caps
K. bich

Dental troubles

HOMOEOPATHY DIGESTIVE & NUTRITIONAL TROUBLES OF THE FIRST INFNACY

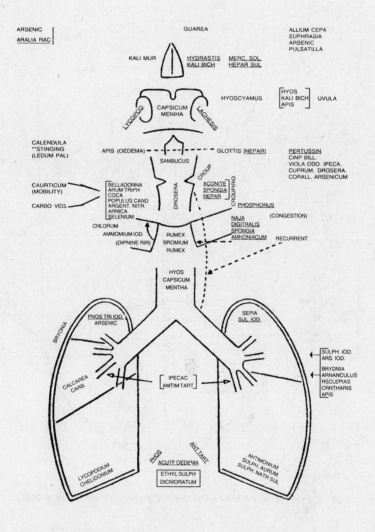

Exported ground Remedies of the Respiratory system with thin satellites.

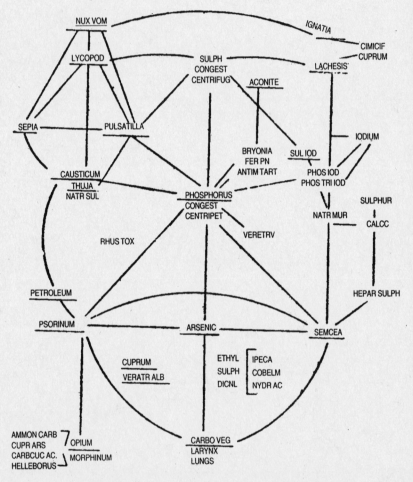

Important ground remedies of the respiratory system with their satellites